PHYSICIANS FOR THE PEOPLE

NEXUS

NEW HISTORIES OF SCIENCE, TECHNOLOGY, THE ENVIRONMENT, AGRICULTURE, & MEDICINE

NEXUS is a book series devoted to the publication of high-quality scholarship in the history of the sciences and allied fields. Its broad reach encompasses science, technology, the environment, agriculture, and medicine, but also includes intersections with other types of knowledge, such as music, urban planning, and educational policy. Its essential concern is with the interface of nature and culture, broadly conceived, and it embraces an emerging intellectual constellation of new syntheses, methods, and approaches in the study of people and nature through time.

Physicians for the People

Black Doctors and the Struggle for Health-Care Equality in Alabama, 1870–1970

JACK D. ELLIS

THE UNIVERSITY OF ALABAMA PRESS
TUSCALOOSA

The University of Alabama Press
Tuscaloosa, Alabama 35487–0380
uapress.ua.edu

Typeface: Scala Pro

Cover image: Twelve of the fourteen Black doctors appointed to the medical staff of Birmingham's Holy Family Hospital, 1954. UAB Archives, University of Alabama at Birmingham.

Cover design: Sandy Turner Jr.

Cataloging-in-Publication data is available from the Library of Congress.
ISBN: 978-0-8173-2223-6 (cloth)
ISBN: 978-0-8173-6186-0 (paper)
E-ISBN: 978-0-8173-9545-2

Contents

Illustrations and Maps

Figures

Maps

Foreword

Jack D. Ellis's *Physicians for the People: Black Doctors and the Struggle for Health-Care Equality in Alabama, 1870–1970* details the trials and tribulations of African American physicians over the course of a century. That inquiry is not pretty. These doctors and their patients suffered time and again. Hospital privileges were denied to Black practitioners, and some white doctors would not treat Black patients. No medical school in the state would teach Black men or women. Black men and women seeking to become physicians needed to leave home and attend one of only two schools that trained Black people as physicians: Meharry in Nashville or Howard in Washington, DC. There was almost no activity that segregation and discrimination did not menace or destroy. Course discriminatory treatment, violent threats, and outrages just because the white power structure allowed for these things do not begin to show the depths of deprivation and despair that African Americans physicians faced.

Yet reading Ellis's book, you cannot come away depressed. It is a story of triumph in some cases, ingenious survival in others. The vignettes that Ellis includes are mesmerizing, transfixing. You hurt deeply for the affronts Black physicians experienced, but then you see the meaning of perseverance. At its rawest, *Physicians for the People* impressively conveys just how committed, wise, and extraordinary the male and female doctors were. It was a monumental battle for them and their patients.

Part of the beauty of the book is the care with which the author constructed his narrative. The book is a collective biography, but it is not just a prosopography. It is a series of individual stories about people doing real things in real time, facing real obstacles. Individual agency often carries the day, although not always. The book is heavily reliant on quotations both from interviews the author conducted and from other sources. You can almost hear the men and women speak. You can sense their frustrations and virtues. Theirs was a labor of love, and the book is a virtual living document of sources and source material that speaks to times both past and ever so present. The narrations are vibrant and poignant. You can see great progress and at the same time realize that very little has changed.

Alabama was a far Blacker place in 1870 than it is now. African American medical men were scarce. That scarcity remains today. By the turn of the twentieth century, Black doctors overwhelmingly took up residence in cities. There they served as apothecaries, small businessmen, and, most impressively, institution builders. Frozen out by the white medical hierarchy, they erected a series of parallel institutions to serve Black medical men and women. Then they went further. Discrimination and segregation exacerbate poverty. Lack of treatment for the diseases that ravaged the mass of poor Black folk in Huntsville, Montgomery, Birmingham, and elsewhere in the state was truly appalling. Black doctors established various clinics to treat the onslaught of patients as expeditiously and effectively as possible.

Not surprising, Black physicians were at the forefront of the civil rights movement and intimately involved in the state's Medicaid debacle. Federal legislation mandated that states partially fund Medicaid and help determine who is eligible. The state of Alabama staunchly opposed Medicaid expansion and hounded physicians who served Medicaid patients in great numbers. Their accounts were audited, and many of the doctors were treated as guilty because of the volume of their claims. Those physicians were overwhelmingly Black, as were their patients. Ellis reminds us that Black Americans have a very different and much poorer health profile than white Americans. He concludes the volume by discussing the Affordable Care Act of 2010.

The Nexus series is dedicated to history that cuts across specialties and approaches. We especially welcome stories about the South. The story of Alabama's Black physicians is clearly a Southern one; segregation and discrimination are the primary movers. We have decided for this important book to broaden a bit what we mean by cutting across specialties. Certainly the book is both a history of health care and a history of medicine. Ellis shows us the medical and professional dilemmas physicians encountered, the skills and training that they possessed, and the incredible odds that accompanied their delivery of health care to their patients. We are proud to have it in the Nexus series.

—ALAN I MARCUS FOR THE NEXUS SERIES EDITORS

Preface

The story of Black doctors in Alabama forms part of a larger narrative in the struggle of African Americans to attain equality. My interest in the topic grew out of earlier research on doctors and the public health movement in France before World War I—specifically, from my efforts to show the links between physical disorders and economic conditions. This theme appears often in the social history of medicine, from Jacques Léonard's study of health and hygiene in rural Normandy and Brittany during the nineteenth century to Edward H. Beardsley's analysis of medical care for Black people and mill workers in Georgia and the Carolinas during the twentieth century. In 1996, the French anthropologist Didier Fassin, a prolific investigator of poverty and sickness in France, Africa, and Latin America, argued that health reflects the distribution of wealth and power in a society, as seen in life expectancy rates, which then stood at seventy-five years for the forty richest nations of the world and at fifty-five years for the forty poorest.[1]

Black Americans have always fared worse than white Americans when it comes to enjoying the benefits of material progress and medical discovery. In his book *The Health and Physique of the Negro American*, published in 1906, the Black sociologist and civil rights leader W. E. B. Du Bois argued that high mortality rates among Black people were rooted not in racial inferiority but in "the conditions of life," a fact illustrated by tuberculosis, which was three times higher among Black people than among white people. Edwin T. Witt, a Black physician from Alabama who spent his childhood in Birmingham's Woodlawn community during the Depression, recalled how the disease was "the scourge of early adolescence" in Black neighborhoods, taking the lives of several of his friends and classmates. When he himself developed a dry cough and chest pain, his mother took him to see a Black doctor in the neighborhood who did a tuberculin skin test: "It was a four plus, meaning the germ had entered my body."[2]

Another case in point is infant mortality, the product of enteritis, pneumonia, whooping cough, and other childhood maladies, as well as lack of prenatal and postnatal care. In their exhaustive study of race, medicine, and health care in the United States, W. Michael Byrd and Linda A. Clayton note that during the first two decades of the twentieth century, the death rate for nonwhite children in the United States was 149.7 per thousand live births, as opposed to 92.8 for white births. Conditions were worse in the South, where in 1937 only 35 percent of Black newborns had a doctor in attendance, as opposed to 90 percent for white people. While a general improvement in health and hygiene during the first six decades of the twentieth century reduced infant death rates, by the mid-1960s they still stood at 38.8 per thousand live births for nonwhite people, as opposed to 20.6 for white people.[3]

The post–Civil War history of African American health care in Alabama mirrors these patterns. For that reason, the lives of its Black physicians, dentists, pharmacists, nurses, and midwives hold special significance, illuminating both the causes for health-care disparities among African Americans and the reasons for their continued underrepresentation in the medical professions. Alabama offers a valuable case study in other ways as well, particularly in showing how culture, geography, and race have historically determined the availability and quality of health care. Its regions were diverse, ranging from Catholic and coastal Mobile to the impoverished counties of the cotton-growing Black Belt, where mortality rates among African Americans remained high throughout the twentieth century. Other regions included industrial Birmingham and Anniston, the isolated and largely white counties of the Appalachian northeast, and the mill towns of the northern and central sections of the state.

At the center of my study are African American doctors who practiced in Alabama between the late 1870s and the civil rights movement of the 1960s. During those years, a total of 241 Black medical graduates passed their licensing examinations and opened offices in the state. I began my research by posing certain questions: What were their geographical and family origins, and why had they been attracted to the study of medicine? Where had they trained, and how did they manage to function as professionals in a climate of racial oppression? What was their relationship to white doctors practicing in their communities, and how did they compensate for their systematic exclusion from local medical societies and hospitals?

In seeking answers, I used three methods. First came the search of available primary sources, ranging from census returns to African American newspapers. Of special significance was the *Journal of the National Medical Association* (*JNMA*), which began publication in 1909 as the voice of the National Medical Association (NMA), founded fourteen years earlier as the Black counterpart to the American Medical Association (AMA). The *JNMA* featured scientific articles as well as news on state and local NMA affiliates, Black hospitals and nursing schools, biographies, and obituaries.

Most useful in identifying Alabama's Black doctors were the annual membership lists of each medical society in the state's sixty-seven counties as they appeared in the *Transactions* of the Medical Association of the State of Alabama (also known by its ironic acronym MASA). This was the official journal of the all-white organization. Here, the names of licensed practitioners who were not members of the association also appeared, followed in the case of Black physicians by the abbreviation "col.," or colored, a routine practice of the era that ceased only in 1965. Typically, entries contained the doctor's name, medical school attended, city and address of practice, and the date his or her licensing examinations were passed. Equally helpful were the records of the State Board of Medical Examiners at the Alabama Department of Archives and History. These contain information on medical graduates applying for licenses to practice in the state and include the names of examiners, test questions, answers and scores, letters of recommendation, and occasionally photographs.

My second step, after collecting and coding biographical information on the 241 doctors, was to create a database using the Statistical Package for the Social Sciences (SPSS). This provided a useful tool for examining a host of variables relating to the doctors' lives and careers. The statistical findings appear throughout the book. Unless otherwise indicated, information for all tables was derived from this database.

A third method was oral history, and early in the research, I decided to place highest priority on completing this phase of the work, owing to the ages and frail conditions of those whom I wished to interview. The resulting oral history collection, which is located at the University of Alabama at Birmingham (UAB), consists of fifty-five interviews with physicians, dentists, and family members who were able to shed light on conditions affecting African American medical practice in Alabama between the 1920s and 1970s. Included are my interviews with fourteen retired professors at Meharry Medical College in Nashville, where two-thirds of Alabama's Black doctors received their training. Other items are my sessions with Sonnie Wellington Hereford III in Huntsville, a 1955 Meharry graduate who became a leader in the city's civil rights movement and whose six-year-old son was the first Black child to enter a previously all-white public school in Alabama. The Hereford interviews formed the basis of our coauthored book, *Beside the Troubled Waters: A Black Doctor Remembers Life, Medicine, and Civil Rights in an Alabama Town*, published by the University of Alabama Press in 2011.

Portions of the edited and condensed oral histories have been integrated into the historical analysis that follows. They include the doctors' recollections of childhood, family life, and early education and their evolving interest in the sciences, which occurred despite the weakness of libraries and laboratories in the Black schools. Next are their memories of medical training and the problems they encountered once in practice, from the wholesale poverty of their patients to the parallel worlds in which Black and white practitioners pursued their calling. Finally, there are the doctors' accounts of the years spent trying to gain admission to Alabama's county medical societies, where membership was required in order to be admitted to hospital staffs and to pursue specialty training. As this book will show, this proved to be the hardest battle of all, despite the fact that Black doctors had passed the same licensing examinations as white doctors.

A collective biography of this kind has the added advantage of permitting us to reflect on broader issues of Black health, as the doctors witnessed them firsthand. Chapter 1, framed against the infamous Syphilis Study and material conditions in the Black Belt, traces the role of Tuskegee Institute in improving African American health and welfare and in encouraging the growth of the state's nascent Black medical corps, despite the violence many of its members experienced at the hands of the Ku Klux Klan. Chapter 2 presents a profile of Alabama's Black doctors, drawn from the database of the 241 individuals and supplemented by oral history, and explores the doctors' early education, their reasons for pursuing careers in medicine, their professional training, and their region of practice. Chapter 3 describes the doctors' patterns of practice and, drawing again on the oral histories, their work as physicians to the poor.

Chapter 4 turns the spotlight on Birmingham and the campaign of African American doctors, ministers, journalists, and business leaders to create a hospital of their own. Though unsuccessful, these efforts helped to produce the Slossfield Health Center, one of the most innovative experiments in Alabama's medical history. These years also saw the first breakthroughs in providing Black physicians an opportunity to practice in well-equipped hospitals—in this case, Catholic facilities, whose creation in the 1940s and 1950s reflected the church's growing social outreach in the state.

Chapter 5 analyzes the role that Black doctors and dentists played in Alabama's civil rights movement and demonstrates how its triumphs helped them in their attempt to break down the doors of county medical societies. The final chapter describes how, despite the gains of the 1960s, the struggle for civil and professional rights remained an unfinished revolution, as white physicians found new ways of maintaining their privileges while evading new civil rights laws. The chapter also describes the implementation of Medicaid in 1970 and how state medical authorities often hounded Black doctors who developed large Medicaid practices, and it concludes with a brief look at the Affordable Care Act of 2010 and the ensuing debate over Medicaid expansion.

From their first appearance in Alabama, Black physicians held out the hand of cooperation to their white counterparts in hopes that they would be allowed to treat their patients in the state's hospitals while refining their knowledge and skills. The gesture was largely ignored. Despite their lofty position as arbiters of scientific medicine and as counsellors to the sick and dying, white doctors tended not only to share the racist norms of their time and place but often to exceed them. As will be seen, the inability of Black doctors to acquire hospital training came at an enormous price to their careers and to the health of the state's Black citizens.

Acknowledgments

Numerous individuals and institutions have helped me in the writing of this book. My colleague at the University of Alabama in Huntsville (UAH), Andrew J. Dunar, then chair of the Department of History, supported my application for a sabbatical leave in order to begin work on the interviews used in this book and over the years was a strong supporter of the project.

Tim L. Pennycuff, associate professor and university archivist at the University of Alabama at Birmingham (UAB), provided invaluable assistance in locating documents and photographs relevant to African American health and medical practice in the state; he also helped to draw up a deed of gift to be signed by each interviewee, whereby the oral histories and transcriptions would be preserved as part of UAB's holdings. The sessions were conducted between 1997 and 2005.

I am indebted to the staffs of the Lister Hill Library at UAB and the Birmingham Public Library, and I owe special thanks to that of the Salmon Library of UAH, which was unfailingly helpful in locating books, articles, and medical journals needed for the work. I mention in particular Gary Glover, Linda K. Vaughan, Elizabeth Rose, Rose Bridgeforth, Michael Manasco, and Charlotte Olson.

In Montgomery, Norwood A. Kerr, archival reference librarian at the Alabama Department of Archives and History, helped me locate medical records containing biographical information on Alabama's Black doctors. Cheryl J. Hamberg, then director of the Meharry Medical College Library in Nashville, and Mattie McHollin, head of the Meharry Medical College Archives, put me in touch with a number of retired faculty at the school and provided space at the library for me to conduct several of the interviews.

My thanks also to A. J. Wright, retired associate professor and director of the section on the history of anesthesia in the Department of Anesthesiology library at UAB, who, on several occasions, shared information derived from his extensive web-based documentation of Alabama's Black physicians before World War I. Linda Bayer Allen, retired from the Planning Department of the City of Huntsville, tracked down several court and probate documents relating to the career of Dr. Harold F. Drake (1922–1979), son of the president of Alabama A&M and a Meharry graduate who began practicing in the city in 1948. My thanks also to John Allison of the Morgan County Archives and to local historian Peggy Allen Towns, author of several books on the Black experience in northern Alabama, both of whom assisted me in locating photographs of Willis E. Sterrs (1867–1921), Decatur's first Black doctor and founder of the Cottage Home Infirmary.

Carolyn A. Eaton, daughter of pioneering civil rights physician Hubert A. Eaton of Wilmington, North Carolina, allowed me access to her father's papers, located in the William Madison Randall Library Special Collections of the University of North Carolina at Wilmington. My work there occurred before I decided to make Alabama the primary focus of my research; nevertheless, reading Dr. Eaton's letters and other documents detailing his battle against racism in the hospitals and schools of New Hanover County, combined with his autobiography, *Every Man Should Try*, published in 1984, formed an important step in my understanding of the African American medical experience in the South. I am indebted to Jerry Parnell, manager of Special Collections, and Luann Mims, graduate research assistant, for their assistance during the time I spent on campus.

I am grateful also to the spouses of Alabama's Black practitioners who assisted me and often had their own fascinating stories to tell. Marguerite W. Franklin, ninety-two years old at the time of our interview, provided valuable information on the life of her husband, James A. Franklin (1886–1972), one of Mobile's earliest Black doctors. Alma W. Foster, who was married to Dr. Maynard V. Foster (1923–1977), shared details of her husband's practice and his successful efforts to eradicate racial barriers in Mobile's hospitals. Geneva Drake Whatley, who held a nursing degree from Meharry and was married to Dr. Drake, recounted her role in her husband's work and the difficulties he faced from the earliest days of his practice.

I owe a special debt to the late Claudia M. Donalson, widow of Dr. Latha M. Donalson (1900–1973), who provided insights about her husband's practice and his small hospital in Fayetteville, Tennessee, which often held Black patients from nearby towns in northern Alabama. Mrs. Donalson also permitted me the use of her husband's Meharry Medical College yearbooks, which contained names, cities of origin, and photographs of numerous Black doctors practicing in Alabama during the 1930s and 1940s. Charlotte Rose Walker, assistant professor of general and oncological surgery at Meharry and daughter of the legendary Black surgeon Matthew Walker (1906–1978), a close friend of Dr. Donalson's, met with me to discuss her father's work at Meharry, where he taught some of the physicians included in this study.

In several cases, family members in Chicago, Cleveland, Detroit, Atlanta, and other cities provided recollections and occasionally documents concerning relatives who had been driven out of Alabama. Charlotte E. Johnson of Alton, Illinois, daughter by a second marriage of Alonzo H. Kenniebrew (1875–1943), the school physician at Tuskegee Institute whom the Ku Klux Klan forced to leave town in 1902 for having treated a white woman, shared extensive information about her father's life, including newspaper clippings and photographs.

Mobile native Ophelia Burnett Northcross—a retired registered nurse living in Detroit and formerly married to Dr. David C. Northcross Jr., son of Drs. David C. Northcross (1877–1933) and Daisy Hill Northcross (1881–1956), both of Montgomery—supplied important details about the Northcross family in Alabama and her own work with Daisy Hill Northcross in Detroit, to which the family fled in 1917. Northcross Jr., eighty-three years old at the time of our interview, shared with me details about the cause of his parents' flight from Montgomery, which followed threats of violence from a local white physician who was outraged over his father's reversal of a medical procedure that the white doctor had performed on a Black patient.

The late Linda Kenney Miller generously shared some of the writings by her grandfather John A. Kenney Sr. (1874–1950), medical director of Tuskegee Institute's John A. Andrew Memorial Hospital, who was hounded out of the state in 1923 by the Ku Klux Klan after he sought to hire an all-Black medical staff at the newly opened hospital for Black veterans. Allison Williams of Saint Paul, Minnesota, helped to fill in some of the blanks regarding her great-grandfather Charles E. Thomas (1863–1933), a physician and drug store owner in Anniston, Alabama, who was periodically harassed by local authorities and murdered by an unknown assailant. Alfreda Swan Wallace of Tuskegee sent me newspaper clippings and answered questions by telephone regarding her father, Dr. Lionel F. Swan (1906–1999), who in 1951 left Birmingham for Detroit after the death of one of his patients who had been denied admission to Jefferson-Hillman Hospital.

Most of all, I am grateful to the doctors and dentists and, in several instances, the spouses of those who practiced during the Jim Crow era, all of whom welcomed me into their homes and shared memories of their lives. They have all since passed on, but this record of their courage and contributions to African American health care will, I hope, preserve their memories and set an example for future generations.

Abbreviations and Acronyms

AAMC	Association of American Medical Colleges
ACA	Affordable Care Act
ACIPCO	American Cast Iron Pipe Company
ACLU	American Civil Liberties Union
ACMHR	Alabama Christian Movement for Human Rights
AMA	American Medical Association
AMDPA	Alabama Medical, Dental, and Pharmaceutical Association
AME	African Methodist Episcopal Church [African American]
ASMA	Alabama State Medical Association [African American]
ASTP	Army Specialized Training Program
CSC	Community Service Committee [Huntsville]
HEW	Department of Health, Education, and Welfare
ILD	International Labor Defense
JAMA	*Journal of the American Medical Association*
JMASA	*Journal of the Medical Association of the State of Alabama*
JNMA	*Journal of the National Medical Association* [African American]
MASA	Medical Association of the State of Alabama
MIA	Montgomery Improvement Association
NAACP	National Association for the Advancement of Colored People

NDPA	National Democratic Party of Alabama
NHA	Negro Hospital Association [Birmingham]
NMA	National Medical Association [African American]
NYA	National Youth Administration
OBGYN	Obstetrics and Gynecology
OEHO	Office of Equal Health Opportunity
PHS	United States Public Health Service
SCLC	Southern Christian Leadership Conference
TVAH	Tuskegee Veterans Administration Hospital
UAB	University of Alabama at Birmingham
UAH	University of Alabama in Huntsville
USA	University of South Alabama [Mobile]
WPA	Works Progress Administration

PHYSICIANS FOR THE PEOPLE

CHAPTER ONE

Tuskegee's Public Health Crusade, 1881–1970

Tuskegee Institute's campaign to improve African American health during the years after its founding in 1881 forms an essential backdrop to the story of Black doctors in Alabama. In order to understand the link between Tuskegee's early leadership in this area and the appearance of Black physicians in the state, we begin by examining the role of Booker T. Washington and his successors in promoting what contemporaries called the hygienic crusade, an idealistic movement that began and continued to grow in the West with the triumphs of bacteriology.

Even after the passage of Jim Crow laws in Alabama and ratification of a new state constitution in 1901 that stripped Black people of the right to vote, Tuskegee clung to its identity as an agent of hygienic reform based on science and the leadership of Black physicians. During a campus speech of 1913, Birmingham's Ulysses G. Mason—who had trained in surgery at the University of Edinburgh and was reputed to have one of the largest Black practices in the South—portrayed doctors as pioneers in the crusade to preserve human life, armed as they were with the discoveries of Louis Pasteur and Joseph Lister and in daily contact with the masses.[1]

Mason's remarks came during the opening of Tuskegee Institute's John A. Andrew Memorial Hospital, named after the Massachusetts governor who had helped create the all-Black 54th Massachusetts Volunteer Infantry Regiment during the Civil War. Funded by a gift of $55,000 from the governor's granddaughter and built with the help of Tuskegee's students, the gleaming colonial-style structure contained fifty-five beds and housed laboratories, x-ray services, a diet kitchen, and convalescent wards. During the dedication ceremonies, John A. Kenney, school doctor and personal physician of Booker T. Washington, expressed hope that Andrew Memorial would become "a hub which will radiate in all directions throughout this community, Macon County, the state of Alabama and the entire South."[2]

Further securing the school's reputation as a center of Black medical culture was the opening of the Tuskegee Veterans Administration Hospital (TVAH) ten years later. Although the TVAH and Andrew Memorial had separate goals and missions, there was considerable overlap, ranging from rotating staff appointments to joint out-patient clinics for impoverished African Americans living in the region. Black doctors outside the state acknowledged Tuskegee's importance, despite its location in a poor, heavily Black county in the Deep South. "Isn't it strange," the *JNMA* asked in 1931, "that the greatest center of Negro medicine and surgery today is not Washington, Nashville, Philadelphia, Chicago, New York, St. Louis, Kansas City—but Tuskegee, down near Big Swamp, in the Black Belt of Alabama?"[3]

Despite its early reputation, Tuskegee's leadership in advancing Black health and welfare has been obscured in memory by the ill-famed Tuskegee Syphilis Study. This longitudinal investigation, launched in 1932, was the brainchild of the United States Public Health Service (PHS), whose white scientists and physicians worked in collaboration with Dr. Eugene H. Dibble Jr., the Black medical director of Andrew Memorial Hospital. It ended only in 1972, after a whistleblower revealed its existence, though penicillin had been available since the late 1940s. The decision of the PHS to allow the disease to run its course in surviving participants has made the study a symbol of medical arrogance and racism. The term "Tuskegee" itself, as historian Susan B. Reverby has rightly observed, has become in popular culture "*the* word for racism, experimentation, and government deceit."[4]

Though morally indefensible, the Syphilis Study does not diminish the achievements of Booker T. Washington, George Washington Carver, and John A. Kenney. The same is true for the contributions of John W. Chenault and John Franklin Hume in the fight against polio, and those of health-care reformers such as Henry W. Foster Jr., who between 1965 and 1973 sought to improve maternal and infant health in Tuskegee and surrounding counties. Though separated in time, these medical pioneers faced a common challenge: how to ameliorate an acute health-care crisis in the region that had been long in the making.

BOOKER T. WASHINGTON AND THE DOCTORS

The first generation of African American physicians in Alabama bore the unmistakable imprint of Booker T. Washington. This can be seen in their views of race relations and in their belief that Black entrepreneurship in the form of pharmacies and infirmaries would strengthen their professional prospects. In a bid to halt lynchings and to improve the worsening economic plight of Black people, Washington had laid out his views in a speech opening the Cotton States and International Exposition of 1895 in Atlanta. There, he proposed a new racial compact whereby Black people in the South would accept the social and political inequality then being codified in Jim Crow laws in return for white support of Black efforts to build schools and acquire industrial and agricultural skills as a path out of poverty.[5]

How this so-called Atlanta Compromise and its emphasis on industrial education played out in the field of medicine tells a more nuanced story. Along with fostering the practices of several Black doctors in Tuskegee and nearby Montgomery, Washington supported plans to create the all-Black National Medical Association (NMA), which came to fruition just one month after his Atlanta speech. Fourteen years later, he provided financial backing for the newly founded *Journal of the National Medical Association* (*JNMA*) and began sponsoring a variety of projects aimed at improving the skills of Black doctors and the health of African Americans. Washington's activities in these areas tend to confirm the positive assessment of his life by historian Robert J. Norrell, who has judged Washington's place in history not by the standards of contemporary Black rivals like W. E. B. Du Bois but by what was possible in Alabama's oppressive racial environment.[6]

To be sure, Washington went out of his way to assure white financial backers that his goal was not to train Black people for the intellectual professions; instead, he stressed the urgency of needing to produce Black workers skilled in agriculture, the industrial trades, and business.[7] Nevertheless, the quest "to make our bodies better fitted for the uses of life," as he once put it, was a recurring theme in his speeches and letters. This can be seen in his observations regarding high death rates among Black people from tuberculosis and other diseases born of poverty and poor housing. He also cited the role of inadequate nutrition, a bitter irony, he said, given the South's agricultural abundance. In a speech at Howard University in 1909, Washington went further, extolling the Black doctor as a missionary whose work in prevention would someday overshadow that of curing diseases. He proposed doubling the number of Black physicians in the

United States, estimated then to be 3,500, in order to achieve a ratio of one per seven thousand Black people.[8]

From his first years at Tuskegee, Washington made numerous efforts to attract Black doctors to Alabama, starting with Cornelius Dorsette. Born in Eden, North Carolina, in 1851 or 1852, Dorsette had been Washington's classmate at Hampton Institute in Virginia and later moved to Syracuse, New York, where he worked as a handyman and chauffer for a white doctor. The doctor encouraged him to pursue a career in medicine and promised him financial support. Dorsette accepted the offer and enrolled at what was then called the University at Buffalo Medical Department, where in 1882 he became the second Black person to receive a degree there.[9]

The following year, Washington wrote to Dorsette, urging him to settle in Montgomery. He noted that more than half the population was Black, that some were wealthy, and that there was no Black doctor in the town. He offered to furnish Dorsette with an introduction to the leading Black ministers, adding, "One co[lored] M.D. in Atlanta is making $2000 a year. Don't see why one can't do as well in Montgomery."[10] Dorsette soon found himself in Alabama, where he succeeded in passing his licensure examinations. He was the second African American in the state to do so, after Burgess E. Scruggs of Huntsville, who in 1879 had completed his training in the Medical Department of Central Tennessee College of Nashville, founded by Methodist missionaries and later known as Meharry Medical College.[11]

Washington offered fulsome praise for Dorsette, later boasting that he was the first Black doctor "to professionally enter the ex-confederate capitol."[12] Despite harassment from some Black followers of a quack named Yellowstone Kit who peddled "liver pads" for the treatment of aches and pains and whose admirers were angered over Dorsette's protection of a Black preacher who had criticized the popular folk healer, the new doctor went on to open a pharmacy on Dexter Avenue, near the capitol. "Since the establishment of this drug store the threats against Dr. Dorsette have completely hushed," Washington said, noting that the drugstore was located on Dexter Avenue, "only a few rods from where Jefferson Davis in delivering his inaugural speech said that he would found a government whose chief corner stone would be slavery."[13]

At Washington's urging, Dorsette took on the task of helping another Black medical graduate prepare for Alabama's licensing examinations, this one a product of the Woman's Medical College of Pennsylvania named Halle Tanner Dillon. Daughter of an AME bishop and sister of the artist Henry Ossawa

Tanner, she came to Montgomery after being offered the job of resident physician at Tuskegee Institute, for which she applied after Washington asked officials of her school to nominate one of its graduates, and she had been the choice. He warned her, however, that she would first have to pass the state boards. It required enormous courage for a Black person, and especially a Black woman, to sit before the Southern white males who made up the examination panels. Some were ex-surgeons of the Confederacy; others were products of the Medical College of Alabama in Mobile, one of whose founders was Josiah Clark Nott, a proponent of pseudo-scientific ideas that regarded Black people as biologically and morally inferior to white people.

In August 1891, Dillon began her ten-day examination, proctored by the state health officer. Three days into her ordeal, she wrote to Washington, assuring him that "if they mark me fairly" she would pass, though she mentioned having been accosted by a policeman in the capitol building who demanded to know why she was coming there every day. On the twenty-third, she reported that the surgery section had been hard but that she thought she did well: "I am so tired at present that I feel when [I] finish my last branch I shall have will power enough to enable me to get back to Tuskegee and that will be about all until [I] have gotten over to some degree the strain which this examination has made upon me both mentally and physically."[14] Three weeks later, Dillon learned that she had passed with an average of 78.81. Her achievement made her the first woman, Black or white, to earn a medical degree in Alabama.[15]

By that time, twenty-eight African American doctors had passed the state's medical licensing examinations and opened practices. These represented only a fraction of the nine hundred or so in the nation, of whom most were located in the South, where the vast majority of African Americans lived. While Alabama's Black population, which stood at 45 percent of the total, seemed to offer good prospects for a Black physician, its harsh racial climate and the widespread belief that the state's licensure examinations were impossibly difficult discouraged many medical graduates from settling there.

As a result, Black doctors in 1890 constituted just 1.5 percent of all physicians in the state, a smaller proportion than in other Deep South states. By 1910, Alabama's Black medical corps stood at ninety-six, of which a third were clustered in Birmingham and its industrial suburbs. Ten years later, the number had grown to 106, who represented 4.7 percent of all physicians in the state. Figure 1.1 shows their actual numbers and how they compared with those in six other Deep South states.

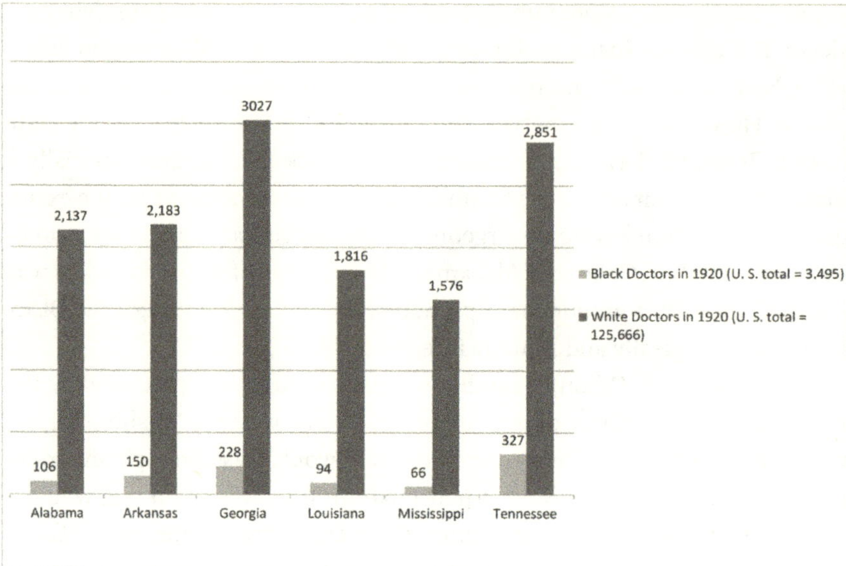

Figure 1.1. Black and white doctors in Alabama and the Deep South, 1920. (Numbers derived from Todd L. Savitt, "Entering a White Profession: Black Physicians in the New South, 1880–1920," *Bulletin of the History of Medicine* 61 (1987): 507–40.)

Except for Mississippi, Alabama's proportion of Black physicians was lower than that of neighboring states and considerably so in relation to Tennessee and Georgia. Tennessee, for example, had developed a comparatively strong African American medical culture, as evidenced by its six Black medical schools. In the end, all but one of the six disappeared; of the fifteen private and denominational Black medical schools that had existed since Reconstruction, only two were able to survive the famous 1910 report of Abraham Flexner for the American Medical Association recommending that schools with poorly trained faculty and inadequate laboratories be closed. The two exceptions were Howard University School of Medicine in Washington, DC, founded in 1869, and Meharry Medical College in Nashville, founded in 1876. Leonard Medical School, a part of Shaw University in Raleigh, North Carolina, which trained 8 percent of Alabama's Black physicians, closed in 1919.[16]

PHYSICIAN-PHARMACISTS AND PHYSICIAN-SURGEONS

In accordance with Washington's encouragement of Black entrepreneurship, the first generations of African American doctors in Alabama generally operated drugstores, which allowed them to fill prescriptions while supplementing their incomes by selling elixirs, cosmetics, magazines, and tobacco. Avoidance of hostile white pharmacists was another motive for their registering with the title, which required only the possession of a medical degree. Although the Alabama Pharmaceutical Association made repeated appeals to the state legislature to tighten its control of them, Black-owned drugstores continued to flourish, each offering a variety of services.

In Selma, Lincoln L. Burwell's drug store sold ice cream, soda water, and coca wine while providing a telephone booth and an office for medical consultations. In Birmingham, the office of Logwood Ulysses Goin included both a drugstore and mortuary. In Decatur, Willis E. Sterrs's Magnolia Drug Store featured a mortuary as well as an ice cream parlor. The latter was of no small importance. Houston Brummit, the physician-grandson of Dr. William H. Brummit in Talladega, has described his grandfather's drugstore as a place "where black mothers could freshen up and sit down with their children to enjoy a dish of ice cream after shopping in the town—a convenience otherwise unavailable to them in segregated Talladega that forbade blacks to share in the amenities available to whites." By serving as a social oasis, Brummit "easily increased his revenues and patient referrals."[17]

We know a great deal about Dr. Brummit owing to his grandson Houston Brummit, who had access to family documents and oral histories, including those of his grandfather's third wife, Olla Brummit. A native of Tallapoosa, William H. Brummit was one of sixteen children of parents born into slavery. After completing his studies at Talladega College, he earned a medical degree from Meharry in 1904, then sat for his licensure examinations, scoring an average of 81.6.[18] Brummit prospered during his early years of practice in Talladega, using his earnings to open the New Era Pharmacy while purchasing prime property downtown. According to Olla Brummit, he was the first person in town to own an automobile, and his house, built on a rise along the highway outside of town, sported a generator, bathroom tiles, and a marble bathtub that made the house a subject of gossip among white and Black people alike.[19]

Similar patterns can be seen in the career of Charles E. Thomas in the mineral-rich town of Anniston, located in the Appalachian foothills of east-central Alabama. Thomas had done premedical training at the University of Michigan, then headed to New York, where he enrolled at the Long Island College Hospital, finishing in 1890. That same year, he took his licensure examinations in Calhoun County, Alabama. Until a law of 1907 consolidated all medical licensure examinations under a single state board, applicants could sit for either state or county boards. Of the seventy-five physicians in this study who received their degrees before 1907, a total of sixty-one took county boards, usually in the area where they intended to practice. That the vast majority chose county over state examinations is unsurprising, given the high failure rates on the latter.[20]

Thomas was a warm admirer of Booker T. Washington and saw Anniston as an excellent place to start. Though the county contained nearly ten thousand African Americans, there was no Black doctor. Moreover, Anniston prided itself as a model industrial city of the South, where Black workers could find jobs in the foundries and cotton mills, a claim that failed to note their position at the bottom of the economic ladder.[21] Despite this, Thomas's practice flourished over the next few years, and by 1894 he had opened The Drug and Medicine Emporium, which was housed in a three-story brick building in the town's Black business district. One contemporary described it as being "splendidly set up" while another praised it as being "one of the best colored drug stores in the state."[22]

An example of how a Black doctor went about adding a pharmacy to his practice can be seen in the case of Dr. Burwell. After graduating from Selma University, he went on to Leonard Medical School, finishing as valedictorian in 1889. Afterward, he sat for the state boards in Montgomery, passing with an average of 81.75.[23] He then opened a practice in Selma, where African Americans formed a majority, most of them living in extreme poverty. In order to purchase drugstore stock, he borrowed from his brother-in-law, only to see the venture collapse within a few months. Deeply in debt, he took matters into his own hands:

> I started again without a cent of money. I went out to a drug store in East Selma and bought three dozen cologne bottles, pints and half-pints, and washed them out myself, and put the labels on myself. And when I went out and saw a patient and the medicine would cost a dollar and a half I would tell him I would send the medicine back to him, and I would go out and buy the medicine and treat him, and if I had another patient with the same disease I would have enough of the same medicine to treat him. And so, I went on, and did not pay anybody till I owed two thousand dollars. I finally had enough to redeem my credit, and now I do not owe anybody.[24]

Included among the oldest members of our group were fifty-one who styled themselves as physician-surgeons. Some had honed their skills in postgraduate seminars at Tuskegee, Howard, or Meharry, while others benefitted from postgraduate training with eminent Black surgeons, among them Chicago's George C. Hall and Ulysses G. Dailey, who often visited Alabama. For most, limited practical experience was obtained only on those occasions when they were allowed to assist white doctors who were operating on patients of the Black doctor in question.

Deprived of training in well-equipped white hospitals, Black doctors sought help wherever available. Contributors to the *JNMA* often offered advice on how the solitary practitioner could obtain the best results when operating in a home—why it was better to lay the patient on a kitchen table covered by an oil cloth rather than on a bed, why reduced side effects made chloroform superior to ether as an anesthetic, or how a simple stew boiler could be used to sterilize instruments. Under such conditions, the dangers of infection were great, but more than a few Black patients were willing to take the risk. In describing how he had corrected a retroflexed uterus at a patient's home, one doctor recalled that "she readily consented for me to do whatever was necessary just so I did not send her to a hospital."[25]

Among the state's most successful Black physician-surgeons was Dr. Sterrs of Decatur, located in northwest Alabama along the Tennessee River. The son of parents born into slavery, he had been awarded one of the few places open to African Americans at the University of Michigan and received his medical degree there in 1888, passing Alabama's licensure examinations with a respectable 79.12 average.[26] Surveying the progress of Black people in America in 1901, the Boston magazine *Our Day* described him as "the most prominent of the two hundred colored proprietors of drug stores in the United States."[27]

By then, Sterrs had opened the Cottage Home Infirmary and Nurse Training School, a two-story building of eighteen rooms. In 1910, the *Pittsburgh Courier*, a Black newspaper, praised the hospital's work, noting that it offered free nurse training to promising young women and that of 150 patients treated over that year, not one died. That same year, the NMA's Committee on Medical Education described the wards at Cottage Home as being "lighted by electricity, well-heated and ventilated." Sterrs himself won praise as "the Superintendent, Physician, and Surgeon-in Chief."[28]

In Talladega, Dr. Brummit was able to improve his surgical talents with the help of Talladega College's president, who made one of its two-story houses on campus available to him. The president then enlisted help from a northern philanthropist named E. A. Goodnow in transforming the house into a modern health-care facility that would serve both students and the Black community. In 1910, the E. A. Goodnow Hospital opened with twenty-one beds and an attached dental office. In addition to performing surgeries, Brummit used the facility to strengthen the college's nurse-training program. As Houston Brummit notes, Goodnow for a time was the sole hospital in Talladega and admitted only Black patients. In an ironic twist, it was the white patients who had to go elsewhere for health care.[29]

In 1912, John A. Kenney estimated that there were sixty Black-owned establishments in the United States bearing the name hospital, sanitarium, or infirmary. Of that total, the NMA singled out just seventeen that merited the name hospital; they included four in Alabama, of which the oldest was Hale Infirmary in Montgomery, having fifty beds and a staff of nine white surgeons assisting the town's Black doctors, who numbered eight. Next, with forty-five beds, was the Tuskegee Institute Hospital, precursor of Andrew Memorial. Goodnow Hospital in Talladega had twenty-one beds and Cottage Home Infirmary in Decatur, twenty.[30]

NATIONAL NEGRO HEALTH WEEK, DR. JOHN A. KENNEY AND THE JOHN A. ANDREW CLINICAL SOCIETY

Among Tuskegee's earliest public health efforts was National Negro Health Week, a community-based idea that had been around since the early years of the century. Projects typically involved the creation of local sanitary committees led by Black doctors, ministers, and others whose task would be the teaching of prevention. In a report to Tuskegee Institute's Board of Trustees in May 1915, just six months before his death, Washington noted the work of his school in helping the Hampton Institute promote what was then being called National Health Week. The idea of a week devoted to public health education, Washington added, was gaining broad support from white physicians, state boards of health, superintendents of schools, the YMCA, the Anti-Tuberculosis League, and white women's clubs.[31]

In Alabama, Washington received support in planning National Negro Health Week from several leading Black doctors in the state, among them the surgeon Arthur McKinnon Brown of Birmingham. As outgoing president of the NMA in 1914, Brown proposed a national Negro health day to be held on the fourth Thursday of each October in all communities that had an NMA member. An honors graduate of the University of Michigan Medical School, Brown stood out for his brilliance early on. According to one account, he chose to practice in Alabama because of the intimidating reputation of its licensure examinations. His scores more than justified his self-confidence: physiology, 100; hygiene, 98; anatomy, 93.75; medical jurisprudence, 93; surgery, 89; obstetrical operations, 86; physical diagnosis, 84; mechanism of labor, 82; chemistry, 79.50; and natural history and the diagnosis of disease, 73.4. His average was 87.8, among the highest ever awarded in the state.[32]

It was left to Robert Russa Moton, Washington's successor, to carry out the work of National Negro Health Week. Until The PHS assumed oversight of the program in 1932, a committee at the school managed the event, choosing a week in early April. It featured presentations on children's health, tuberculosis prevention, eradication of flies and mosquitos, and community activities aimed at cleaning up houses, pigsties, stables, and privies. Although National Negro Health Week failed to address the structural causes of the health crisis afflicting Alabama's Black population, it helped to promote hygienic education, lasting until 1951 and spreading to 2,200 communities in thirty-two states. Of special importance were the local clinics it sponsored—a total of 750 in 1936, for example. With the help of both Black and white physicians, these clinics offered smallpox vaccinations, tuberculin tests, and preschool physical examinations.[33]

In addition to these public health activities, Booker T. Washington devoted considerable efforts toward strengthening the NMA. At its first meeting in Atlanta in 1895, the organization had adopted no constitution or bylaws and met only twice over the next eight years, attracting just fifty or so members. Starting with a meeting at Meharry in 1903, the group began holding annual conventions for the reading of papers. A turning point occurred five years later when, with a membership of around three hundred and financial support from Tuskegee Institute, the NMA's executive board agreed to create the quarterly (later bimonthly) *JNMA*. Serving as associate editor and business manager was John A. Kenney. Born in Virginia, Kenney was an honors graduate of Hampton Institute and had trained at Leonard Medical School and Freedmen's Hospital before coming to Tuskegee. There, he expanded the mission of the school hospital to include not just students but all members of the local Black community. Starting in 1904, Kenney also served as general secretary of the NMA. Four years later, he became editor-in-chief of its journal, a position he would hold for the next thirty-two years.

Dr. Kenney enjoyed strong support at Tuskegee Institute, which strengthened his influence nationally. Black practitioners "had no more loyal supporter than Booker Washington," he wrote in later years, recalling how, in the wake of criticisms voiced during a meeting of the school's executive council regarding the cost of the NMA's journal, Washington called him aside to reassure him: "Don't pay any attention to them. As long as you wish to have that Journal published here, it will be done."[34]

In August 1912, Tuskegee Institute hosted the annual meeting of the NMA, which elected Kenney as president for the upcoming year. Attended by two hundred Black doctors, the meeting was notable for its free clinics on behalf of Macon County's rural Black families, many of whom streamed onto the campus aboard wagons and carts to find treatment for tuberculosis, syphilis, malaria, heart disease, and pellagra. In all, the clinics treated over five hundred patients and performed twenty-five operations, ranging from tonsillectomies and appendectomies to removal of uterine fibroids. "The scene around the Institute Hospital every morning beggars description," one observer wrote. "Men with face tumors, others with hare-lips, women suffering from abdominal tumors, mothers with deformed children, all waiting for charity treatment."[35]

In 1918, Kenney devised a tool for better coordinating the planning of the clinics. This was the John A. Andrew Clinical Society, which started off with twenty-six members whose ranks included several of the best-known Black surgeons in Nashville, Birmingham, Atlanta, and Chicago. A third of the founding members were Black doctors practicing in Alabama, among them Henry Clay Bryant and Ulysses G. Mason of Birmingham, Alfred D. Simington of Mobile, Lincoln L. Burwell of Selma, Charles E. Thomas of Anniston, and Willis S. Sterrs of Decatur.[36]

Soon, Kenney began extending the clinics from three days to a week, and, in an effort to broaden interracial contacts, he asked prominent white surgeons and specialists to participate. The clinic held in April 1921, for example, attracted 126 attendees and included participants from The Johns Hopkins Hospital, Massachusetts General, and the medical faculties of Harvard and the University of Illinois. Kenney later boasted that because Black doctors could not attend postgraduate courses at the schools the white attendees were a part of, "we brought these institutions to them."[37]

Subsequent meetings drew smaller numbers but continued to be impressive: seventy-nine in 1922, sixty-four in 1923, and sixty-eight in 1924, the latter representing Black and white doctors from eighteen states, mostly in the South. In a speech to the NMA years later, Kenney claimed that "fully one-half or more of the Negro medical men in this country have attended this Clinic and at least twenty thousand patients have been treated there." Among Black physicians in Alabama who received their licenses before 1931, over a third had attended one or more of the annual meetings at Tuskegee.[38]

Both Kenney and Washington understood the professional isolation in which the great majority of the state's Black doctors worked and lent the school's support to a fledgling effort to create an Alabama affiliate of the NMA. Among the most outspoken advocates for the idea was Dr. Sterrs of Decatur, who served as the NMA's secretary-treasurer. He took the first step in creating a Black medical society in the state, becoming, in the words of a colleague, the *accoucheur* of the Alabama Medical, Dental, and Pharmaceutical Association (AMDPA). The group met first in 1896, but subsequent gatherings were sporadic and poorly attended, many potential members no doubt fearful of associating themselves with an organization known for promoting the economic interests of Black doctors. The AMDPA's best showing came at its Birmingham meeting of 1910, when it managed to attract seventy Black doctors, dentists, and pharmacists.[39]

The group managed to keep going for a few more years, meeting in tandem with the NMA's annual conference in Tuskegee in 1912, 1916, and 1920. The death of Dr. Sterrs in a fishing accident in 1921 robbed the organization of its most effective leader, but his efforts had helped to convince a significant number of his colleagues to join the NMA. While just ninety-four of Alabama's Black doctors before 1970 are known to have joined the NMA, membership levels were highest among the earliest generations—47 percent for those receiving their medical degrees in 1921 or earlier, as opposed to 29 percent for those graduating after 1921.

Meanwhile, three city-based Black medical organizations tried to pick up some of the slack. In Birmingham, Arthur McKinnon Brown and the dentist Joel A. Boykin organized what came to be known as the Mineral District Medical Society. Black doctors in Montgomery and Mobile followed suit, creating, respectively, the Capital City Medical Association and the Mobile Medical, Dental and Pharmaceutical Association, later renamed the Gulf Coast Intra-Medical Society in an effort to include colleagues from coastal Mississippi. Nevertheless, these groups remained largely dormant during the 1920s and 1930s, dependent on a just a handful of members willing to organize meetings.

PERSECUTION AND FLIGHT

Dr. Kenney's advocacy on behalf of Black physicians inevitably enraged white supremacists in the state. Their threats could not be ignored: between the end of Reconstruction and World War II, thousands of African Americans died of lynchings in the United States, 340 of them in Alabama alone. Leading the onslaught was the Ku Klux Klan, which attracted widespread support in the state and included several prominent white doctors purported to be members. By 1925, the Alabama Klan had grown to 115,000, and the intensity of its violence set it apart in the nation.[40]

Kenney's trial by fire came in 1923 during the opening of the Tuskegee Veterans Administration Hospital (TVAH). The government's plan had been to consider both Black and white candidates for the medical staff, but objections from Tuskegee's white leaders caused the Veterans' Bureau to back down. In January 1923, the bureau announced a plan to hire exclusively white personnel, having already named a Southern segregationist as director. In a meeting with President Warren G. Harding, Moton sought support for at least partial Black staffing, and soon a new head of the Veterans' Bureau began recruiting Black employees who had the requisite civil service credentials. These measures provoked a firestorm of white opposition in Tuskegee and throughout the state.[41]

When the hospital began operations in June, it did so with an all-white staff, though the Veterans' Bureau promised that positions would be filled by Black personnel as soon as qualified candidates could be found with experience in the treatment of tubercular and psychiatric patients. In response, the NMA urged members to suggest appropriate names, noting that there had been no greater unity among Black people on a single issue since Reconstruction.[42] In a meeting between officials of Tuskegee Institute and a delegation of white residents from the town, the latter threatened to burn the campus down if Moton and Kenney did not withdraw their support for an all-Black staff. Both stood their ground, marking them for death threats from the Klan.

White outrage flared even brighter in late June after several Black nurses began working at the new facility and after the Veterans' Bureau announced that thirty-three Black doctors had been added to the civil service list of eligible practitioners. On July 3, an estimated one thousand Klan members traveled by automobile from Montgomery to Tuskegee, then drove in silent procession through the streets of town and past the grounds of Tuskegee Institute before burning a forty-foot cross on Dr. Kenney's lawn. Within twenty-four hours, Kenney sent his family North; he himself followed a few days later and settled in New Jersey, where he went on to found the Kenney Memorial Hospital in Newark.[43]

As passions cooled, the Veterans' Bureau moved quickly to hire Black applicants for lower-level positions at the TVAH. Then, in August, six Black doctors joined the staff, three of whom had trained in psychiatry and one in physical medicine and rehabilitation. Three months later, Eugene H. Dibble Jr., a Howard graduate who had come to Tuskegee to train under Kenney shortly before Klan threats forced Kenney to flee, performed an appendectomy at the TVAH, the first operation done there by an African American. Soon, almost 90 percent of staff positions were held by African Americans, including twenty-one doctors and dentists.[44]

Kenney's flight from Tuskegee represented just one of many examples of the harassment suffered by Alabama's Black practitioners both before and after World War I. These, in turn, were part of an upsurge in attacks on Black professional and business elites across the country, symbolized by the murder of Dr. A. C. Jackson during an assault by white mobs on African Americans in Tulsa in 1921. In his study of Black physicians during the Jim Crow era, Thomas J. Ward Jr. notes how some doctors were run out of town for being too "uppity," while others suffered beatings at the hands of sheriffs and policemen. In the summer of 1918, a Black physician in Vicksburg, Mississippi, named John A. Miller, a medical graduate of the University of Michigan, was tarred and feathered.[45]

Finding oneself in the Klan's crosshairs was not an uncommon experience for Black doctors. Threats came not only from uneducated white people but occasionally from white colleagues who were quick to react with anger to any perceived lack of professional deference. Just two years after Dr. Kenney was forced out of Tuskegee, a Black physician named John Wesley Darden, who had built an extensive practice in the town of Opelika in east-central Alabama, experienced such white indignation firsthand.

The trouble started after Dr. Darden's younger brother, Walter Theodore, who had just completed his medical training at Howard, arrived to join him in his practice. One day, the younger Darden encountered an African American boy with a broken arm and only a bandage to stabilize it and promptly made him a cast. When the white doctor who had misdiagnosed the fracture discovered what Walter Theodore had done, he called John Wesley Darden in a fury. Soon afterward, a cross was burned on the lawn of Darden's home, and he decided that his brother had to leave town. He arranged for him to practice at the Newark, New Jersey, hospital that Dr. Kenney had created.[46]

An earlier case involved David C. Northcross, an 1881 graduate of the University of Illinois College of Medicine who had built a successful practice in Montgomery's Black community. Like Dorsette, Northcross had married into a prosperous Black family—that of Daisy Hill, daughter of a truck farmer named William Hill. Born into slavery, her father had started off peddling fruits and vegetables in the post-emancipation years while buying cheap land on Montgomery's outskirts. Over time, he acquired sufficient wealth to give his children a Northern education. Daisy Hill enrolled at Temple College in Philadelphia, where, according to her future daughter-in-law, Ophelia Burnett Northcross, her light skin enabled her to pass for white. She finished in 1902, then came home to teach elocution at the State Normal School for Colored Students.

In 1909, Daisy Hill married Dr. Northcross, and the couple began laying plans for a small hospital attached to their home to be known as the Northcross Sanitarium. To maximize profits, Dr. Northcross suggested that she return North and earn a degree in medicine. She soon won admission to Loyola University School of Medicine in Chicago, where she completed her training in 1913. The following year, Daisy Hill Northcross passed the Alabama boards, becoming, at that point, Alabama's only Black female practitioner.

According to his son, Dr. Northcross served on the staff of Hale Infirmary and had gotten to know the white doctors who treated their own Black patients there. His relations with them were at first cordial, but that changed in 1916 when he decided to reverse a bowel resection performed by a white surgeon on a Black male, who had afterward come seeking Northcross's help. The operation, known as a colectomy, removed part of the patient's large intestine and included a colostomy, wherein the colon is attached to the skin to allow removal of waste. Northcross judged the surgery unnecessary and reestablished the colon and bowel. When the white surgeon found out what he had done, he flew into a rage, vowing to tar and feather Northcross. The latter decided to leave the city, and Daisy Hill Northcross followed soon after the birth of their son. Settling in Detroit, the two worked as a team to build a practice, creating the first privately owned Black hospital in the state.[47]

Even worse than questioning a white doctor's authority was treating a white woman, as Mobile's James A. Franklin knew firsthand. A graduate of Lincoln University in Pennsylvania, Franklin completed his training at the University of Michigan in 1914. Learning of the need for a Black doctor in Conecuh County, Alabama, northeast of Mobile, he moved with his family to Evergreen, the county seat, where he began doing house calls on foot. Drafted soon after American's entry into the European war, Franklin discovered that he had little hope of becoming an officer, despite the need of medical care for Black draftees. While he and one other Black physician from Texas received commissions in the Medical Reserve Corps, they never got orders to report and were instead assigned duty as privates in the hospital corps of Camp

Zachary Taylor in Louisville. Franklin's second wife, Marguerite W. Franklin, remained forever embittered: "They called him into the army, and they wouldn't consider him as a doctor in the army. Yet he had to wait on the people just as if he was a doctor."[48]

Discharged in 1919, Franklin returned home just as the global influenza pandemic was starting to gain a foothold in tiny Evergreen. A midwife named Thelma Shamburger, who lived in a Black section of North Mobile known as Africatown (named after the enslaved West Africans who were brought there illegally in 1860 aboard the ship *Clotilda*), was just nine years old when Franklin showed up at her house, asking her father if he could rent a room. "A gang was mad at him 'cause he doctored a white lady," Shamburger recalled later, noting that the woman's husband had managed to get Franklin out of Evergreen on a southbound train.

In later years, Marguerite Franklin related what her husband had told her about the incident: "They had a bad siege of flu at that time, and this white man had a Negro woman working for him, and all of the [white] doctors turned [his wife] down, said that they couldn't cure her. So [the Black woman] told him, 'If you want to be cured, you get Dr. Franklin. He'll cure her 'cause he cured my daughter from the flu.' So the white man did. He called Doctor. And Doctor cured the lady. And the whites ran him out of there."[49]

Being perceived as an abortion provider was still another source of danger, as in the case of Anniston's Dr. Thomas. His troubles began in 1908 with an office visit by a Black woman named Onether Crawford, who was suffering from "flooding," or excessive bleeding, which sometimes occurs during the menstrual cycle or the first trimester of pregnancy. According to a witness, Crawford's first of two consultations occurred on a Friday evening, at which time Thomas prescribed medication for her bleeding. Judging from later testimony, the substance was an alkaloid-based drug known as ergot. Derived from the fungus of rye grain, ergot in small doses was a common treatment for menstrual bleeding. In higher doses, it could cause uterine contractions and miscarriages.

Crawford's condition worsened overnight, and she returned the next morning. According to Thomas's accusers, it was during this second visit that he used surgical instruments to induce an abortion, a charge that he denied. After her second visit, Crawford suffered a miscarriage and sought help from a white surgeon in town named Thomas Jefferson Brothers. After examining her, Brothers reported that he had found a "rupture in the neck of the womb" that could have been produced only by childbirth or by surgical instruments.

A complaint was filed against Thomas, and a grand jury returned an indictment. The charge was that he had violated section 4305 of the Alabama Code of 1896.[50]

Thomas's trial took place before an all-white jury, which found him guilty of inducing an abortion. Sentenced to three years in the state penitentiary, he filed an appeal based on the vagueness of the indictment. Two of the seven justices on the appeals board agreed, finding fault with the judge's decision to excuse Onether Crawford from testifying, which precluded a cross-examination. A majority, however, upheld the verdict. The fact that state medical authorities made no effort to strip Thomas of his medical license seems to underscore the weakness of the case against him. In fact, the Board of Pardons released him after just five months.

In Talladega, Dr. Brummit's downfall was occasioned by rumors that he had treated white women. If true, it was only one of many instances in which he flirted with danger. The town's white doctors were certainly aware of his surgical skills as well as his high standing among the state's Black physicians, which was confirmed in 1924 when members of the John A. Andrew Clinical Society chose him as president. But Brummit's knowledge and reputation could not protect him when conflicts arose with local white doctors.

On one occasion, Brummit accused a white surgeon named Clarence E. Salter of stealing one of his patients. On another, he accused an elderly physician named Edward Bates Wren, who had allegedly whipped a Black female servant, of lying when he placed the blame on the servant. Equally damning were reports that in talks to churches and fraternal orders, Brummit had urged Black farmers to protect their economic interests; in particular, he had criticized the practice of storing their cotton in white-owned warehouses until cotton prices went up, which resulted in exorbitant rental fees.[51]

Houston Brummit's description of what happened to his grandfather shows the perils awaiting those who did not keep their place. On the night of May 7, 1924, several carloads of white men abducted Brummit at gunpoint from his home, bound and blindfolded him, and drove him to a dense spot of woods fifteen miles outside town. After charging him with having practiced medicine on white women and warning him that he had ninety days to clear up his affairs and get out of town, they stripped him and beat him with a whip until he passed out. The *Chicago Defender* described the assailants as being unmasked and counting in their ranks some of the leading members of the community. None was ever arrested, however, and Brummit soon sold his New Era Pharmacy and went to Chicago to prepare for the

Illinois medical boards, working as an assistant to other Black doctors until he could build his own practice. What he suffered in Alabama, the *Chicago Defender* said, "has done more than anything else to stimulate a northern migration from this vicinity."[52]

Of the 241 Black physicians who practiced in Alabama before 1970, 23 percent are known to have left the state, which represented a significant loss of heath care for the state's African Americans. The doctors' departure mirrored Black migration as a whole: between 1900 and 1940, Alabama lost roughly 20 percent of its Black population to the cities of the North and Midwest, part of the 1.8 million African Americans who left the South.[53]

CONDITIONS IN MACON COUNTY AND THE BLACK BELT

Driving the efforts of Tuskegee's leaders to improve the lives of African Americans were the appalling health conditions in Macon County, where the town is located. In the rural areas, access to either a Black or white doctor was extremely limited, as was true for the Black Belt as a whole. Figure 1.2 shows the number of white and Black inhabitants per white physician in the seventeen counties of the region, which in 1950 held just over a third of the state's Black population. Russell County, bordering Georgia to the east, had just one white physician per 6,727 inhabitants of both races. In Lowndes County, the figure was one per 6,005.

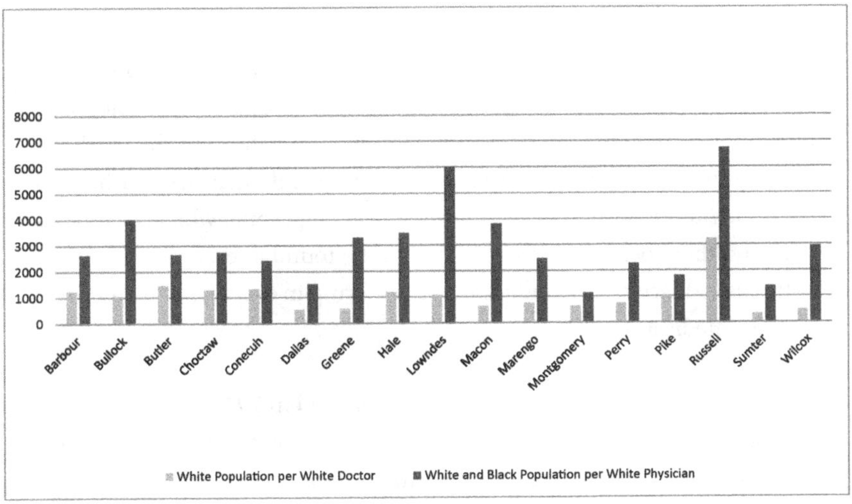

Figure 1.2. White and Black populations per white physician in Alabama's Black Belt counties, 1950. (US Census data and Transactions of the Medical Association of the State of Alabama, 1950.)

Haunted by slavery, the stretch of dark, rich soils and cotton plantations in the Black Belt ran across the south-central portion of the state into Mississippi and included such cities as Selma, Montgomery, Tuskegee, and Union Springs. In the latter, where Black residents outnumbered white residents four to one, a white medical graduate of the University of Virginia named Seale Harris, later to acquire fame for his work on diabetes, reported in 1902 that the majority of Black residents were "poorly fed, improperly clothed, and their houses . . . located on the lowlands of the suburbs of the town, where all the dampness of the atmosphere predisposes them to tuberculosis and where all the filth and impurity of the town drain directly into their wells and streams, contaminating their only source of water supply." Harris noted that in Bullock County, home to Union Springs, the average annual death rate for Black people was 31.17 per 1,000, as opposed to 11 per 1,000 for white people. Tuberculosis alone accounted for 20 percent of all Black deaths in the town.[54]

Macon County itself stood as a depressing portrait of how poverty had ravaged the bodies of Black people, something that Halle Tanner Dillon discovered soon after assuming her duties as school physician at Tuskegee Institute in 1891. In a report to the alumnae association of the Woman's Medical College of Pennsylvania three years later, she described what she had witnessed, noting that great numbers of Black people, unable to afford the two-dollar-per-mile fee of white doctors, had simply resigned themselves to a life of suffering and premature death:

> In the vicinity of our school are hundreds in need of medical attention, children with tubercular tendencies, sore eyes, various skin troubles, and in a pitiable condition generally. Women with faces bearing the marks of pain upon them: faces which testify but too plainly that life is a burden with such diseased bodies. In the miserable log-cabins which are dotted here and there over the county, will often be found a fever-tossed patient, with flushed face and bounding pulse, suffering in every fiber, but entirely without medical aid."[55]

In his classic *Shadow of the Plantation*, published in 1934, a Black sociologist at Fisk named Robert S. Johnson described Macon County as a place where "the shell of the past hangs on in the agricultural economy" and where the lingering effects of slavery were reflected in the high numbers of Black famers working land owned by someone else. He and his researchers studied 612 Black families in all; his investigation revealed that during the year prior to his study, just

258 of the 612 Black families surveyed had visited a physician. All but one of the physicians were white, several of whom owned plantations. Before agreeing to provide treatment, they often demanded that the family pledge something of value, such as a cow or a mule, in case the fee was not paid. Because a home visit could cost as much as twelve dollars, Black families often treated their own ailments, relying on herbal and folk remedies and an assortment of patent medicines, including the purgative Black Draught, a cold and fever treatment called White Wonder Salve, and quinine for malaria.[56]

An eyewitness to the health crisis in Macon County was a Black doctor named William H. Frazier, a Baltimore native who had earned a degree in medicine from Howard in 1927. He had completed an internship at Andrew Memorial and then sat for the Alabama boards, earning scores between ninety and one hundred in all fields.[57] After marrying a dietician at the TVAH, he opened a private practice in town and over the next five years treated Black patients from Tuskegee and neighboring farms and villages. A man of great cultural attainments, Frazier had an agile mind rooted in the kind of analytic methods used by his older brother, the famed sociologist Edward Franklin Frazier.

As part of his practice, the younger Frazier volunteered to serve as physician for the Black schools of Macon County. During the summer of 1934, he began working with teachers and officials at the county health board in conducting a survey of 632 pupils enrolled in three of the schools. One was in the village of Chehaw, and the other two were in Tuskegee itself—the Washington Public School, located two miles from Tuskegee Institute, and the Lewis Adams School, which was located on campus. The latter, whose pupils belonged to families that were at a higher economic level than those in the other schools, invariably did better on the survey, which Frazier regarded as proof that sickness reflected one's economic conditions.

The survey consisted of questionnaires filled out by the teachers, who recorded the age, weight, and height of each child. Frazier also conducted physical and dental examinations of all 632 children. Finally, he collected blood and stool samples that were then sent to the State Board of Health to identify the presence of such diseases as syphilis and hookworm. The following year, Frazier published the results of his investigation in *Opportunity: A Journal of Negro Life*, published by the National Urban League.[58]

Frazier presented a bleak tableau of the health of Black children in rural Alabama. Using scientific indices for comparing their physical and nutritional status, he reported that 58.7 percent of the children were underweight, 54 percent had dental defects, 22.1 percent had enlarged tonsils, and 48.7 percent had enlarged lymph nodes. Twenty-one percent were found to be anemic—that is, at 70 percent hemoglobin and below on the Tallquist hemoglobin scale. The presence of anemia in so many of the students, Frazier said, had to have a common etiology, which was "marked nutritional derangement."

A subset of questions among 157 older students revealed the absence in their diets of foods rich in calcium, phosphorus, vitamins, and other items having "hemoglobin producing value." Less than half the students, for example, drank milk daily, about the same proportion reporting that their families owned cows, though not all of the cows were productive. Less than half consumed eggs at least three times a week, and though they occasionally ate apples and peaches, their daily intake was deficient in fruits. Instead, grits and rice were the mainstays of the children's diet.

The laboratory samples collected by Frazier found syphilis in 9.6 percent of the individuals tested, a "relatively low rate," he said, when compared with the 36 percent discovered during a syphilis demonstration project in 1930 that was overseen by the PHS in collaboration with the Rosenwald Fund, a philanthropic effort created in 1917 by Sears magnate Julius Rosenwald. The conflicting findings, Frazier said, showed "how variable the incidence of the disease is among different groups of Negroes. The selectness of the group and the better educational contact partly explain the difference in this instance."

Many Black residents of Macon County had looked favorably on the demonstration project, which had performed serological tests for syphilis and administered injections of neoarsphenamine, a derivative of arsenic and a standard treatment for the disease before penicillin became available. It had also provided typhoid and smallpox inoculations as well as diphtheria immunizations.[59]

With so fertile a field of inquiry, the PHS decided in 1932 to launch a full-scale study of untreated syphilis among Black males in Macon County. A total of 399 individuals were selected, to which was later added a control group of 201 who were given simple medications under the guise of curing what was called "bad blood." Without being told the nature of their illness or that they were subjects in a medical experiment, participants were promised medical care, periodic physical examinations and hot meals, transportation to and from Andrew Memorial Hospital, and burial insurance—the latter on condition that they agreed to autopsies.[60]

BLACK PHYSICIANS AND THE TUSKEGEE SYPHILIS STUDY

Until it became public knowledge in 1972, few Black doctors in the state seemed aware of the syphilis study at Tuskegee. Even Fred Gray, the Black attorney who filed a class-action lawsuit that year on behalf of its subjects, recounts in his memoirs how, despite practicing law in Tuskegee and representing Macon County in the state legislature, he had never heard of the study until the story broke.[61] Internist Calvin R. Dowe, who did a residency at the TVAH during the 1950s and stayed on part time while maintaining a private practice, recalled his own surprise: "I hadn't seen the papers. A guy asked me at the filling station why did we doctors let this happen. Let what happen? I didn't even know what he was talking about. We were here. Nobody had let us in [on it]. The physicians who were practicing, seeing people, did not know anything about this study."[62]

Other practitioners responded in similar fashion. The Brooklyn-born polio expert John Franklin Hume, the nation's second Black board-certified orthopedic surgeon who joined Tuskegee Institute in 1949, recalled hearing of the syphilis project only in 1969, when representatives of the PHS appeared before the Macon County Medical Society, of which the Black doctors in the county had only recently assumed control: "They came over and told us that the patients that they were following had not received treatment. And these people had had a positive serology. And they didn't say anything about withholding [future] treatment. They told us what was going on, and we said, 'Well, you know, if this is what's going on by the public health department, there's nothing we can say.'"[63]

Montgomery surgeon Calvin R. Johns Jr., who completed a residency at the TVAH between 1963 and 1968, performed physical evaluations of some of the aging participants but knew nothing about the study:

> I wasn't told anything. But I was a member of the staff, and these guys came back. They told us they had syphilis, and they were being examined to find out what their status was. They ran them through a few blood tests, which I had nothing to do with. Mine was physical assessment of these fellows. I didn't know that this whole thing was going on until after it was exposed. I thought it was a horrible situation for people to deny an individual the right to get treated when knowing full well what the end stages of this disease were.[64]

Those who did have knowledge included a coterie of Black physicians and school administrators, among them Robert Russa Moton, who gave his consent for the PHS to use Andrew Memorial and its staff to carry out the work. Dr. Dibble most certainly understood the study and did all in his power to support it, believing it to be an extension of his school's mission. Though a compassionate man, any ethical concerns over how the PHS intended to proceed seemed curiously lacking. Nor could he have failed to understand the racist features of an experiment focusing solely on Black men, whose deaths were reported promptly to him by members of the then all-white Macon County Medical Society so that autopsies could be performed at Andrew Memorial.[65]

Susan M. Reverby has shown that numerous interns performed routine tasks required of the research, including x-rays, painful spinal taps, and autopsies. As time passed, additional Black medical personnel gained knowledge of what was going on. One was William B. Perry, who operated a mobile "bad blood" clinic, seeking to test for early stage syphilis in rural Black residents. Another was Dr. Reginald James, who had been part of the Rosenwald Fund's earlier demonstration project and in 1939 accepted an offer from the Alabama Health Department to direct the mobile treatment bus.[66]

Accompanying James was Eunice Rivers, a 1922 graduate of Tuskegee Institute's nursing program. Aware of her work in educating rural midwives, Dibble recommended her as an assistant for the study; her duties involved keeping track of the men, driving them to and from the hospital for examinations and tests, and persuading them to agree to spinal taps. When a participant died, Rivers faced the additional challenge of obtaining consent from the family to perform an autopsy. "More than any other single person," Fred Gray wrote, "Nurse Rivers was to personify the Tuskegee Syphilis Study to the six hundred men who became involved in it." Yet when Gray filed a class-action lawsuit in 1973 on behalf of the study's subjects, he excluded her from the list of defendants, describing her as "a lone African American female" in a project conceived and implemented by white physicians.[67]

In her study of Black doctors at the TVAH, Mary Kaplan suggests that the social status of Tuskegee's Black physicians may have led some of them to endorse such research as the Syphilis Study, which used poor sharecroppers as guinea pigs.[68] That some middle-class Black doctors looked down on the masses is indeed probable, as was practitioner prejudice based on skin color. For those who felt its sting, the latter was a particularly insidious form of discrimination. At age ninety-four, Hattie Swope, a Black ex-sharecropper in rural Lawrence County, recalled the injury she still felt over a seemingly minor event during her teenage years involving Dr. Sterrs, who had ignored her when doling out free ice cream to her lighter-skinned companions on their visit to his drugstore in Decatur.[69]

Nevertheless, to assume an equivalence of moral culpability between Black practitioners who knowingly or unknowingly participated in the study and the white public health officials who planned and controlled it is to ignore the many forms of coercive power that federal, state, and local medical authorities had at their disposal. The most powerful actors in the drama were the white medical men of the PHS, some of whom regarded the illiterate Black patients who crowded into the rural clinics they conducted as less than human.[70]

Historian Susan L. Smith has argued that many Black doctors who knew of the study and supported it did not regard it as unjust but as a way to attract greater federal interest in Macon County's health problems, which would enable Tuskegee Institute to continue helping Black people. It was only in later years that the deceit permeating the project came back to haunt them. In an interview conducted by Smith in 1989, the highly regarded public health expert Paul B. Cornely of Howard University said, "I was there and I didn't say a word. I saw it as an academician. It shows how we looked at human beings, especially Blacks who were expendable."[71]

JOHN W. CHENAULT AND THE INFANTILE PARALYSIS CENTER

In 1939, Dr. Kenney returned to Andrew Memorial and for the next five years took up his old jobs as the hospital's medical director and as secretary-treasurer of the John A. Andrew Clinical Society. Under his leadership, the annual meetings stayed true to their original mission, even with the loss of younger physicians to military service during World War II. In 1944, a total of three hundred physicians and surgeons descended on the town, examining six hundred patients and performing one hundred operations. That year, Kenney estimated that since their inception, the annual clinics had treated between fifteen thousand and twenty thousand patients.[72]

Soon after Kenney returned to Tuskegee, the school began focusing on the polio epidemic that had erupted during the 1930s. The effort was headed up by John W. Chenault, a Wyoming native who held a medical degree from the University of Minnesota and trained in orthopedic surgery at the University of Chicago and the University of Iowa. In 1937, Tuskegee Institute hired him as head of orthopedic surgery at Andrew Memorial and as director of its modest twelve-bed unit for children who were disabled. His first step was creation of the Crippled Children's Service, the term then used to describe handicapped infants and adolescents. The work relied on funding from the Rosenwald Foundation and the Children's Bureau and was one of four such centers in Alabama operating under the aegis of state health authorities and the Department of Education.

By 1940, Chenault had examined hundreds of Black children. While 20 percent were diagnosed with polio, others bore marks of the harsh conditions facing the very young in rural Alabama. Ten percent, for example, owed their infirmities to injuries suffered after falling into fireplaces or outdoor fires built for the heating of wash-pots. Another 10 percent had birth injuries caused by poor obstetrical care.[73]

The orthopedist John Franklin Hume, who succeeded Chenault in 1949, recalled in his oral history that at the time there was no place in the South where Black children could be treated. This neglect persisted despite high levels of Black participation in the March of Dimes (the popular name given to the National Foundation for Infantile Paralysis) and in President Roosevelt's famous "Birthday Balls," which were aimed at creating an endowment for the polio treatment center at Warm Springs, Georgia, where the president, who was diagnosed with polio at age thirty-nine, often retreated.

Warm Springs did not accept Black patients. Of hospitals willing to do so, Hume said, most provided little care: "Because of segregation and because of the horror associated with the disease, the nurses were scared to treat Black patients, and whatever hospitals they were put in, they had to go to the basement, and nursing care was given by relatives."[74] Some medical authorities even suggested that Black people were immune to polio. Alleged differences between Black and white susceptibility were rooted not just in misdiagnosis of the disease but in racist assumptions about the Black body, specifically in regard to the "primitive" nature of the Black physique as opposed to the more delicate frame of the white physique. These racist stereotypes persisted despite Chenault's urgent plea to the medical profession "to dispel the appalling indifference so frequently encountered among my colleagues."[75]

Tuskegee's Infantile Paralysis Center, led by Dr. Chenault, opened in January 1941, following a campus visit by President Roosevelt, no doubt aware of growing anger among African Americans over their exclusion from Warm Springs.[76] Roosevelt was also a close friend of the attorney Basil O'Connor, who in 1938 had created the National Foundation for Infantile Paralysis in order to raise money for Warm Springs. "O'Connor was the chairman of the board of directors of Tuskegee Institute," Hume recalled, "and he knew about Chenault, and he knew about the medical problems here, and he knew about the role of Dibble and Booker T. Washington. And because of the pressure for the March of Dimes to do something about the treatment of Blacks and polio, O'Connor selected Tuskegee, because of the medical facilities, to build a unit, which was supposed to be comparable to Warm Springs."[77]

Polio treatment facilities in Tuskegee were housed in a three-story brick building connected to Andrew Memorial Hospital. During the center's first four years, a total of 101 children were admitted there for "after-care," which included medical and surgical treatments, physical therapy and massage, and muscle reeducation aimed at restoring mobility. Chenault's staff consisted of a physical therapist, a head nurse, four graduate nurses, and a technician charged with making braces and shoes. The unit featured a green-tiled basement pool equipped with hydraulic lifts and containing twelve thousand gallons of water heated to a temperature of ninety-two degrees. There were arm and leg whirlpool baths, electro-therapeutic machines, rooms for fitting shoes and braces, and iron lungs for children whose paralysis rendered breathing difficult. About half the children were from Alabama and neighboring Georgia, their families paying according to their circumstances and the severity of the case.[78]

The number of those treated in the Infantile Paralysis Center does not reflect its greater role in research and in the training of Black physicians, nurses, and physical therapists in the care of polio patients. Tuskegee nursing students, for example, spent three of their thirty months of required work there. Dr. Hume, who became interim head in 1949 and later permanent head after Chenault accepted a position in Florida (Hume remained on the job until the Salk and Sabin vaccines rendered the center unnecessary), also stressed its importance in developing new surgical techniques.[79]

HENRY W. FOSTER JR.'S EFFORTS TO IMPROVE INFANT AND MATERNAL HEALTH

Among later Black doctors who struggled to better health conditions in Tuskegee and surrounding areas was Henry W. Foster Jr., who in 1958 completed a medical degree at the University of Arkansas, where he was the only African American student in his class. After interning in Detroit, he spent two years as a medical officer in the Air Force, followed by residency training in surgery at the Malden Hospital in Boston and in obstetrics and gynecology at Meharry. Starting in 1965, Foster spent six months of his residency at Andrew Memorial, where his performance was so exemplary that even before he had completed his training, Dr. Dibble, then medical director, had asked him to stay on.

By that time, Andrew Memorial had grown to 175 beds with a medical staff of ten doctors and two residents, their specialties ranging from surgery, urology, and orthopedics to internal medicine, obstetrics and gynecology, and physical medicine. Embracing a broad mission of training doctors, nurses, dieticians, physical therapists, and social workers, the hospital provided help to the region's rural doctors and midwives when complications arose during deliveries. It also sponsored a variety of free out-patient activities, including prenatal, postnatal, and well-baby clinics and, in 1958, a tumor clinic offering pap smears to test for cervical cancer.

The TVAH had likewise grown in size under Dibble's direction while retaining its primary emphasis on the neuropsychiatric disorders of Black veterans. By the time America entered World War II, it was caring for over 1,700 patients with a staff of 31 physicians, 5 dentists, and 115 nurses. The 1950s saw the introduction of new residency programs in medicine and surgery and later in radiology, ophthalmology, and oral surgery and periodontology. By 1962, ninety-seven Black physicians had completed at least one year of internship and residency training at the TVAH, fifty had done two years, and forty-one had done three.[80] Alabama's Black doctors counted ten who did internships at the TVAH (and an additional twelve at the John A. Andrew Memorial Hospital), plus four who finished three-year residencies at the TVAH.[81]

Eager to work in an environment where he could make a difference in the lives of patients, Foster accepted Dibble's offer, becoming the only obstetrician in an area comprising eight heavily Black counties.[82] During the eight years that he worked at Andrew Memorial (he left in 1973 to become head of obstetrics and gynecology at Meharry's Hubbard Hospital), he devised new procedures for treating the women who visited the hospital, such as improved protocols for cases of preeclampsia and eclampsia. At the suggestion of a nurse named Thelma Walker Brown, and with help from the TVAH laboratories, he also began screening newborns for sickle cell disease, which made early treatment possible for those whose blood samples showed the telltale crescent-shaped red blood cells.

Foster's most far-reaching accomplishment was his successful application for a Maternity and Infant Care Projects grant under Title V of the Children's Bureau. The grant allowed him to create a regional system of rural clinics aimed at reducing high infant mortality through prenatal and pediatric care while also treating diabetes and heart disease.[83]

Not all white doctors in the six-county region were enthusiastic about the clinics, which they feared would cut into their profits. Members of the Bullock County Medical Society, for example, declined Foster's offer to use leftover grant money to create a satellite clinic in their area. Because their approval was required before any federal money could be spent, this left the poorest of the county's ten thousand Black citizens without access to health care.

What turned things around was the election of attorney Fred Gray to the state legislature in 1970. The day after his victory, Gray received a visit from a white businessman who confessed that he had not voted for him but who now offered his services. Gray told him about Dr. Foster's problems in securing approval from the Bullock County Medical Society for a clinic. "I assured him that the program would not interfere with the local doctors' practices," Gray later wrote; "It would not take any money from their pockets because the people who would be treated at the clinic did not have money to pay a doctor."[84]

A few days later, the society gave its approval. The ensuing work of Foster left a lasting mark among local inhabitants, who long remembered "Dr. Hank" for the countless hours he spent driving the backroads of the region, delivering hundreds of babies and sometimes repairing botched abortions. Thelma Walker Brown, the nurse with whom he worked at Andrew Memorial, later told a journalist for the *Los Angeles Times* that the women Foster treated were "the poorest of the poor. Women who didn't have anything." Sometimes, she said, midwives would bring in their premature babies: "I mean, they'd put those babies in boxes with hot water bottles and bring them to us and ask us to save their lives."[85]

In 1970, Foster won election as president of the Macon County Medical Society, replacing Luther C. McRae Jr., one of three white doctors still in town. McRae was a Georgia native who had trained at the University of Florida, and for a time he maintained good relations with Foster, even seeking his advice on difficult obstetrical cases. That changed when Foster and the Black physicians who now controlled the county medical society thwarted a plan by McRae and the other two white doctors to obtain federal money for building a new hospital to replace the deteriorating county facility, which would have allowed them to avoid sending their patients to Andrew Memorial.[86] Defeated, McRae moved his practice to Mount Vernon, Georgia, but the matter was far from forgotten.

More than two decades later, after President Bill Clinton had nominated Dr. Foster to be US surgeon general, McRae tried to torpedo the nomination, asserting that despite Foster's claim of having heard about the Tuskegee Syphilis Study only in 1972, he had attended a briefing of the Macon County Medical Society three years earlier at which two officials of the PHS had informed members of the study, and Foster had voiced no objections. Strangely, McRae could not remember whether PHS officials had told the doctors that treatment was still being withheld for the men in the study, and, as no minutes of the meeting could be located, he was unable to substantiate his claim that Foster was even present. On the contrary, using records from the Alabama Bureau of Vital Statistics, which recorded dates and times of all deliveries on birth certificates, Foster was able to show that at the time of the meeting, he was performing a cesarean section.

In the end, Foster's nomination never made it to the full Senate, owing mainly to his pro-abortion stance. Still, the accusation that he had known about the Tuskegee Syphilis Study and failed to object to it cut him to the quick, standing as it did in contrast to his life of service. As he later wrote, "I couldn't understand how anyone would have thought we would have turned our backs on the very community we had come to serve."[87]

CHAPTER TWO

Becoming Doctors

Who were the Black physicians who practiced in Alabama during the Jim Crow era? While they exhibited a diverse assortment of personalities, attainments, and levels of wealth, they shared many traits in common. Except for ten who hailed from the West Indies and eleven from the North and Midwest, our doctors were mostly products of the South, especially the lower South. Fifty-six percent were Alabama natives, about half of them from counties having majority Black populations. Thirty-four percent of those born in the state had grown up in cities, an experience that brought to them several advantages, from the presence of an urban Black culture to the availability of better schools. At the opposite end of the scale were those from rural areas or towns under three thousand, who represented 46 percent.

An analysis of the occupations of both the fathers and mothers of Alabama's Black doctors before 1970 shows a variety of social levels, though parents who enjoyed comparatively high degrees of economic well-being tend to stand out. Figure 2.1 shows how the fathers of our doctors made their livings. Agricultural trades dominated all other occupations. A quarter of the fathers working the land appear to have owned their own farms; others were listed in census records as tenants, day laborers, and wood cutters. Despite the drive for land among Black people that had marked the post-Reconstruction era, sharecropping with unpaid family labor became the rule for most, the result of predatory practices among white encroachers. These practices came in many forms, from unfair tax assessments to developers who used the absence of wills and the proliferation of Black claimants as a toehold for gaining access to Black holdings.[1]

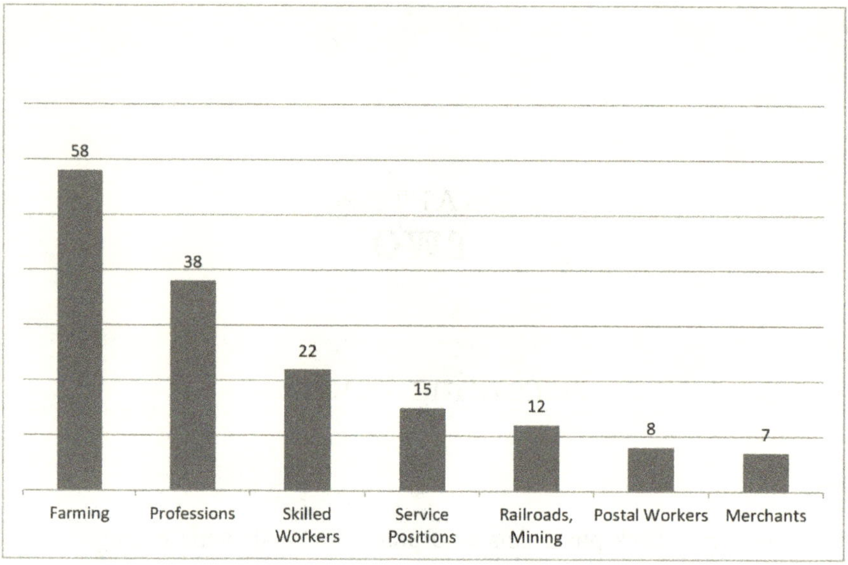

Figure 2.1. Occupations of fathers of Alabama's Black physicians, 1879–1970 (N=160)

Oral accounts suggest that parents or grandparents who succeeded in retaining ownership of their land often owed their success to collective purchases made with family and friends. In Hale County, for example, located in the Black Belt, Charles E. McGruder recounted how his mother was born on land then owned by her family, who later lost it. His father, on the other hand, was born on the family farm and lived there all of his life: "The property that the McGruders owned went all the way down to the Greene County line. There were six brothers involved in this, and the full size of the property was 320 acres." Land ownership conveyed psychological as well as material benefits: "I never felt inferior to anybody, because when I was growing up, we were living on land that belonged to my daddy and his brother. So the feeling was you can always come back home."[2]

In Montgomery, two Black doctors benefitted from an even larger enterprise in collective land acquisition. One was a graduate of the Woman's Medical College of Pennsylvania named Hagalyn Seay Wilson, who opened a practice in the city in 1957. Wilson was the daughter of civil rights leader Rev. Solomon S. Seay Sr. and the cousin of John H. Winston Jr., who began his surgery practice in 1964 after completing a residency at the TVAH. Wilson and Winston were the children of two sisters whose grandparents, during the 1880s, had joined twenty or so relatives and friends, all former slaves, in purchasing a thousand acres of a place once known as the May Plantation, which lay along the Old Wetumpka Highway. The resulting all-Black community, inspired by Booker T. Washington's ideas of self-sufficiency, became known as Madison Park, named after the great-grandfather of Wilson and Winston. The two doctors maintained a lifelong identification with the community, whose elementary school provided teaching jobs for both their mothers. It was also one of the state's first Rosenwald schools, named after the part-owner of Sears, Roebuck and Company in Chicago, who would go on to fund four hundred others in Alabama out of a total five thousand in the South.

Middle-class pursuits such as teaching and the ministry likewise stand out among the fathers' occupations, followed by health-care professionals—five doctors, one dentist, and one pharmacist. The paucity of physicians suggests the weakness of family traditions in medicine at this point, as was true also for dentistry. In 1940, the number of Black dentists in the country stood at just 1,471, of which 48 percent were located in the South—roughly one Black dentist per fourteen thousand Black inhabitants. Alabama had just thirty-eight, which amounted to one Black dentist per twenty-six thousand Black inhabitants.[3]

Fathers belonging to the ranks of skilled workers included barbers, masons, and a scattering of carpenters, shoe makers, metal workers, blacksmiths, and upholsterers. There were also miners, railroad firemen and brakemen, grocery store owners, insurance agents, and postal carriers. At the bottom were several in service positions, from cooks, porters, and chauffeurs to gardeners, janitors, and peddlers.

The oral histories sometimes allude to frequent changes in the occupations of the fathers, not surprising given the unsteady market for Black labor. The father of ophthalmologist Alexander Lee Brewer, for example, taught school in the Wiregrass town of Ozark in southeast Alabama before moving to Birmingham to work as a mail carrier. Finding his salary inadequate to support a family of six during the 1920s, he turned to peddling fruits and vegetables from a horse-drawn wagon, joining scores of other African Americans who dominated the city's peddling trade. Young Brewer and his siblings worked as "jumpers" who would go door-to-door selling baskets of produce, returning to their father with cash in hand. "When I would work on the wagon," Brewer said, "he would give me my share of sales, and as the years passed, he sorta had a truck farm on the side."[4]

Although less is known about the mothers of our doctors, census reports provide important clues. Of 139 known cases of the mothers' occupations, close to 70 percent are listed as homemakers, a designation that obscures their contributions to the family's economic well-being. In some cases, such contributions included shared management of the farm. "There was no question *ever* about who was in charge in the house," McGruder recalled; "It was 'Mother Dear'—and [then] my daddy." While his father knew his multiplication tables and could read the Bible, "boys didn't get a chance to go to school. When a boy got big enough to help around the farm, he began to do chores like helping haul wood or fixing a pasture or clearing new ground, and those things interfered with his going to school. So the girls went to school more than the boys."

McGruder could often overhear his parents discussing plans for the family late into the night: "My mother had gone to college a little bit in order to be able to teach school before she got married. Daddy—I don't know how far Daddy went to school. Mother was good at planning and organizing stuff. I was the oldest child, and the house was very small. So I could hear the discussions going on when [falling] asleep. She'd come up with bright ideas, and, of course, they would agree on it. And then he would go out to do what *they* had decided."[5]

Of twenty-three mothers who worked in middle-class professions, most were elementary or secondary school teachers, along with an additional two serving on the faculties of Black colleges. Those who chose teaching careers faced formidable obstacles, starting with inferior facilities and low salaries. In his classic *Negro Education in Alabama* published in 1937, Horace Mann Bond, father of future civil rights leader Julian Bond, described the gross deficiencies in Alabama's rural Black schools, where in 1930 only 5.8 percent of children of high school age were actually enrolled. Bond noted that in nine Black Belt counties where African Americans formed a majority in 1930, there was not a single Black four-year public high school. That included the state capital of Montgomery, home to more than thirty thousand African Americans, plus an additional twenty-two thousand living in the county. In Alabama as a whole, per capita spending for teachers' salaries per Black child was $4.48, as opposed to $14.39 per white child.[6]

Especially discouraging for Black women pursuing teaching careers was the lack of opportunities for educational advancement. A study of those teaching in thirteen states in 1940, most of them in the South, showed that while the overall percentage who finished four years of college stood at 35.1, for Alabama it was 18.1 and for Mississippi, 9.1.[7] James T. Montgomery, the Birmingham internist who in 1963 became the first Black doctor to win admission to the Jefferson County Medical Society, remembered that his mother went through the eighth or ninth grade: "She had lived with an Uncle James, who was very interested in education back in the teens. And she came up [to Birmingham] to Miles College—they had a high school at that time—and went to high school. At that time, [teachers] could teach in elementary school after finishing the eighth or ninth grade, and she taught there for many years."[8]

Montgomery's father, who had managed to complete only the third grade, worked as a farm laborer in Atmore, northeast of Mobile. Facing hard times, in 1936 the family moved to the Roosevelt community of Homewood in southeast Birmingham, where the father opened a grocery store. There, young Montgomery attended Rosedale High School, where his uncle, a fervent believer in education, was principal. The latter's views were important to Montgomery's development, but his mother was "the one who pointed all of us to get as much education as possible."[9]

Mothers appearing in the oral histories are often depicted as possessed of deep inner strength. Birmingham internist Tyree James Barefield-Pendleton, who had grown up with his mother and grandfather on a sharecropping plot near Natchez, Mississippi, remembered that his mother, Susie Barefield, "had a lot of race pride" and "was very aggressive for that day and time." That included speaking up to white people. One incident stood out: "I must have been about twelve years old, because my grandfather died when I was nine, and this was after his death—[she] was in the store buying a shirt for me. The owner of the store says, 'What's that boy want to be when he grows up?' She said, 'He says he wants to be a doctor.' He told her, 'You better teach him how to plow.' She said, 'Well, he said he wants to be a doctor, so we're gonna try to help him.'"[10]

Hagalyn Seay Wilson often heard stories of her paternal grandmother, who "led the cotton row, led the singing in the cotton field, led the prayer meeting. When the man who ran the store[11] didn't give her gifts that she thought were suitable for her children's Christmas, she began to decide how she could change this situation. She planted vegetables that she could sell on the streets of Montgomery. She raised chickens and sold the eggs, and she never went to the store again for gifts for her children at Christmastime."[12]

LIFE IN THE BLACK SCHOOLS, COLLEGE TRAINING

McGruder remembered his father and mother as being determined to provide the best schooling possible for their children. When he was in the fourth grade, his parents decided that the one-room school he and his siblings attended was inadequate and that they would transfer them to a better one thirteen miles away. The problem was transportation: "They had a bus to take the white kids, but not for the Black kids. The only way you could go to school after you got past the sixth grade was to move down there and live with somebody or get there the best way you could." To solve the problem, his father and uncles combined parts from two dilapidated Model-T Fords sitting out in the car shed so that one of them would run, then built a bus made out of wood and managed to attach it to the vehicle.[13]

By the time McGruder was ready for high school, his father had found work in a steel mill in Fairfield, near Birmingham, to help tide the family over during the Depression. Young McGruder enrolled in Brighton High School, confident that he was now in a place that could provide the quality education he craved. One day, he made an unsettling discovery: "I saw a copy of the list of the books that they used in the Jefferson County schools. A lot of the things they were teaching the white students, they didn't even teach to us." At Brighton, there was no chemistry laboratory, no gymnasium: "There wasn't a typewriter on this high school campus. In 1942, that's when I finished, there was no typewriter."[14]

It was the same in other Black high schools across the state. In Huntsville's Councill School, Sonnie Wellington Hereford III remembered science being taught solely out of a book: "There was no physics lab or biology lab, and what passed for a chemistry lab had maybe seven or eight test tubes, two or three Bunsen burners and beakers, and half a dozen reagent bottles."[15] In Birmingham's Rosedale High School, young Montgomery managed to get a solid grounding in mathematics but finished in 1943 with a shaky foundation in the sciences: "We had work in biology and chemistry and physics, but we never had any laboratory to work in. You did the work just basically from a textbook."[16]

The most fortunate students were those enrolled in laboratory schools (22 percent), which operated under the auspices of teacher-training programs in Black colleges and usually included grades one through twelve. Fully accredited, these schools provided support for students showing an interest in teaching, medicine, and law, and compared with white schools, a much higher percentage of their graduates went on to college. Typical was Jefferson Underwood Jr., who attended the lab school at Alabama State in Montgomery: "I started there in first grade. I went from first grade all the way through. Just about everybody in my class went to college. It was just something we were expected to do. You didn't wonder whether you were going to college or not."[17]

Despite conditions in the Black schools, the fact that significant numbers of their students went on to successful careers suggests hidden strengths. These derived in large part from the teachers, the majority of them women who worked hard to develop the students' knowledge and self-esteem. Many teachers, for example, incorporated bits and pieces of Black history into their classroom materials whenever the opportunity presented itself. McGruder loved these moments: "The schools were segregated, so whenever they felt [like] it, the teachers would talk about Black history. If they felt like telling you something good about somebody who went before us, they would talk about it." Sometime during the 1930s, his teachers organized a class trip: "I went to Tuskegee and saw Dr. Carver before he died. That was one of the greatest things that ever happened to me when I was a boy. I went into Dr. Carver's laboratory and watched him there."[18]

Classroom instruction might also incorporate stories of Alabama-born sports figures like Joe Louis, who in 1938 avenged an earlier loss to the German fighter Max Schmeling by knocking him out, and Jesse Owens, hero of the Olympic Games in Berlin two years earlier. World War II provided other examples. Ninth-grader Sonnie Wellington Hereford III, taking a half-year course called Negro History at Councill School in Huntsville, recalled being surprised one day when his teacher brought her husband to class. He was a Tuskegee Airman home on furlough: "He stood there wearing an officer's uniform, and I shall never forget it. We'd seen mainly privates and corporals among Black people, and now, standing in front of us, was a Black first lieutenant of the United States Army Air Force."[19]

Although the precise number of individuals in our group who earned college degrees is unknown, it is safe to assume that during the first decades after their appearance in Alabama, the proportion was small. In 1910, the AMA's *Flexner Report* noted that while entrance requirements at Howard were "a high school education or its equivalent," those at Meharry were "less than a four-year high school education."[20] During the 1920s, both schools began tightening their entrance requirements. Applicants to Meharry now had to have at least a year of premedical training, which in a few years was increased to two years. Specifically, they needed twelve semester hours of organic and inorganic chemistry, eight of physics, eight of biology, plus six to twelve hours of English composition and literature and six to twelve of a foreign language. Howard, which boasted a larger budget and faculty than Meharry, started the process earlier, and by 1928, 70 percent of its entering class had completed four years of college.[21]

Of the 121 individuals in our group for whom information is available,

60 percent completed their undergraduate degrees at private liberal arts institutions. At the top of the list, and in similar proportions, were Talladega College, Howard University, Lincoln University, Tuskegee Institute, Morehouse College, Fisk University, and Selma University. The rest were products of public colleges, including Alabama A&M, Alabama State, and similar public schools in other states. Of the 121, 36 percent did college study in Alabama; an additional 9 percent earned undergraduate degrees at Howard before entering its medical school, while 8 percent studied at Lincoln College in Oxford, Pennsylvania, which is often credited with having produced a fifth of all Black physicians in the United States before the 1950s.

A student's selection of a college reflected a broad range of goals and motives. Cost and location were usually the most pressing considerations, though family pressures also came into play. In Mobile, the future dentist Lawrence E. Carroll found himself being pulled in different directions. He had three uncles in the dental profession, one of whom pressed him to choose Morehouse; in opposition were Carroll's principal at Dunbar High School and the principal's wife, who lived next door and were both Talladega alumni. Added to those favoring Talladega were two other alumni, Escous B. Goode, one of Mobile's most prominent Black physicians, and his brother, the dentist Plesant W. Goode, both of them close friends of his father's. In the end, Carroll chose Talladega.[22]

For others, the religious preferences of parents played a significant role. Following his graduation from Birmingham's Industrial High School in 1938, Dodson M. Curry enrolled at Johnson C. Smith University in North Carolina, a Black Presbyterian school—a choice that reflected his mother's deep faith. Hagalyn Seay Wilson attended Livingstone College, also in North Carolina and affiliated with the AME Zion Church, the denomination in which her father had trained for the ministry. It was an all-Black college at that time, she said, "five hundred students. Everybody knew everybody. The president knew all the students well enough to make comments as he passed you in the morning on your way to class. The teachers were very caring, and there was a lot of one-on-one teaching."[23]

Among other reasons for choosing a college were thoughts of how one would fit in and what the other students would be like. Before his financial straits forced him to enroll at Alabama A&M, which was near his family's farm, Hereford had planned to attend Tennessee State in Nashville, where he thought he would find a congenial atmosphere for someone of modest origins like himself. By contrast, Fisk "was expensive and was looked upon by a lot of my friends as uppity, by which I mean the students seemed to be mostly lawyers' and doctors' kids from up North."[24]

Fear of being judged as inferior to graduates of elite Northern Black schools haunted others as well. James T. Montgomery, who enrolled in Morehouse College in 1943 after one of the professors came to Rosedale High School looking for students, found it rough going at first: "It was a very difficult transition from high school, where you made a lot of good marks but didn't learn very much." He remembered English as being the most difficult course: "The kids who came down from Chicago, New York, North Carolina, they'd been to better schools. They were better prepared, and it made the first semester and probably the first year very difficult. But after that, we got on a level playing field."[25]

Those in our group who were enrolled in the lab schools typically continued at the same institution for their college training. For some, the thoroughness of their high school studies, and the fact that many of their new classmates had attended poorly equipped Black schools that left them unprepared for college, meant that graduates of the lab schools went unchallenged. John H. Winston Jr., who graduated from Alabama State in 1949, sailed through his courses in chemistry and biology while in college but found himself unprepared for medical school. "We had the basics that other kids didn't have in high school," he said. "When the kids came from other areas in Alabama, they had nothing. I was so far in front of them I didn't have to study. I could just go on my high school experience."[26]

Graduates of Alabama's Black high schools often found themselves struggling in college, the result of having learned science without adequate laboratories. Moreover, the colleges themselves sometimes had to scramble in order to provide premedical training. When Hereford showed up at Alabama A&M in the fall of 1949 asking to take premedical study, the best his advisor could do was to place him in its division of education as a "special student." Soon, Hereford discovered that the biology laboratory contained only three or four microscopes, along with a few test tubes and petri dishes. With encouragement from a biology instructor named Mary Chambers, he managed to master the subject matter and by the end of his first year had earned superior grades in biology, chemistry, and mathematics.

At that point, Hereford applied to Meharry and, to see what would happen, to the University of Alabama Medical School, writing the word "Negro" in the space asking for the applicant's race. Unsurprisingly, the University of Alabama turned him down. Meharry accepted him, contingent on the satisfactory completion of his second year of premedical study, which included three quarters of general physics, three quarters of organic chemistry, and advanced biology, mathematics, and English. Hereford finished with a straight-A average. That, plus a satisfactory performance on the Graduate Record Examination and the Medical Profile Test, ensured that he would become one of six Black students from Alabama in Meharry's class of 1951, which totaled sixty-five.

THE DECISION TO ENTER MEDICINE

As in the case of selecting a college, choosing a career in medicine sprang from a variety of personal motives. Individuals who headed off to college during World War II sometimes enrolled in premed programs as a way to avoid, or at least to delay, serving in what some called "the white army." James T. Montgomery made no effort to hide the fact: "At Morehouse, I found out if you studied medicine, you had a chance to become premed [and] to get exempted from going into the army, because at that time, you could go to medical school, if you were lucky, after spending two years in college."[27]

McGruder, on the other hand, knew that he wanted to be a doctor by the time he was in high school: "I never did exactly know why. That's just what I decided I wanted to do. I was always aiming at being something that would lift me way up above most folks." All this was easier said than done: "I recall when I was a boy down on the farm that the greatest things were these: you could be a sleeping car porter [or] you could be a farm demonstration agent. Then, I had an uncle who was a house painter, and I even got a book and read how to mix paint. I was just gonna do something."[28]

The limited range of opportunities open to African Americans was evident to observers at home and abroad. In *An American Dilemma*, the classic 1944 study of race in America, the Swedish economist and sociologist Gunnar Myrdal reported that the number of Black people in professional, managerial, and white-collar occupations in the United States stood at just 254,000. While this figure had increased by three-fourths between 1910 and 1930, the proportion for white people had undergone similar growth, leaving Black people still in a position of relative inferiority. Slightly more opportunities were available in medicine, Myrdal added, noting that the number of Black doctors and dentists had grown from 3,677 to 5,712 during those same years.[29]

As for law, Black people had far less representation, accounting for only 0.77 percent of all lawyers in 1930, even though the actual number of Black attorneys had increased by one-fourth since 1910. When future civil rights leader Arthur D. Shores gained admittance to the Alabama Bar in 1937, he was Birmingham's only Black attorney. By 1949, there were four and by 1961, eleven, several of whom spent much of their time pleading civil rights cases.[30] Unlike medicine, where one practiced almost exclusively within the Black community, law required constant interaction with white judges, juries, and attorneys who often made little effort to disguise their racism. James T. Montgomery recalled how his uncle, the principal of Birmingham's Rosedale High School, encouraged him to study law rather than medicine, telling him of Black doctors he had seen working as redcaps in the train stations of Chicago. When Montgomery enrolled at Morehouse College, he had intended to follow his uncle's advice but soon changed his mind: "The outlook of the time didn't look too bright for Blacks who were going into law. You'd still be a 'boy' in the courtrooms in Alabama."[31]

The oral histories show that for many in our group, an interest in medicine stemmed from an early aptitude for science. As a seventh grader, Hereford became intrigued by the test tubes and medicine dropper brought to school by a classmate who owned a chemistry set and who showed him how to make clear solutions turn red or blue. A fascination with biology soon followed. Hereford's older brother later described him as "a boy who'd get out there and plow in the sun all day long and talk biology up and down the rows."[32]

Barefield-Pendleton had a similar awakening. After moving to Vicksburg, his mother insisted that he complete his studies at Magnolia Avenue High School, where she made him repeat a biology course he had taken earlier in a poor rural school. He remembered the principal, a man named Bullock, as being a bit "pushy" but also as always encouraging him: "Math was my favorite subject until I got to chemistry, and then chemistry became my favorite subject. Science came easy to me. When I was in chemistry, I could just spread out an equation and tell you what was going to be on the other side. That was almost in my head, whereas other students would struggle with it."[33]

Barefield-Pendleton found inspiration from a Black doctor in Natchez named Albert W. Dumas Sr., who owned a drugstore and clinic and sometimes treated his mother. Similarly, Hiram B. Moore, who would someday treat patients in his hometown of South Pittsburg, Tennessee, and in the small neighboring communities of northeast Alabama, idolized a local Black doctor named William J. Astrapp: "I used to wish that I was a doctor 'cause, see, my mother passed away when I was young, and Dr. Astrapp was her doctor, and he'd come, and he'd do what he could for her. And I used to think about being a doctor way before I was in grammar school. But I didn't see no way I could hardly be a doctor.[34]

As one who commanded respect in the community, a Black doctor was often a figure of awe in the eyes of children. In Anniston, the mother of David Satcher, future US surgeon general, often related to him the story of a Black physician named Fred D. Jackson, who came to the family farm during the early 1940s to treat her son for whooping cough and pneumonia. Dr. Jackson saved young Satcher's life, his mother told him, and he resolved to follow in his footsteps.[35]

An almost legendary Black doctor in Birmingham named Pierce S. Moten helped generate an interest in science for future pediatrician Eugene T. Witt. The victim of tirades and threats from a father addicted to homemade whiskey and increasingly violent, young Witt began spending time with his maternal grandmother. When he was six years old, she caught pneumonia, and Dr. Moten came to visit her every day. Witt found himself mesmerized by the doctor's stethoscope, which piqued his curiosity and eventually his interest in science.[36]

In some instances, it was the absence of a doctor that helped stimulate a child's interest in medicine. An example is Anniston's John William Sherrer, who grew up in Ohio hearing stories from his parents about the trials of finding medical care in rural Bibb County, Alabama, where his father worked as a coal miner: "They migrated to Dayton mainly because when my mother was pregnant with the fourth baby, they couldn't get a physician. She almost died. My father decided he would move North, and he always taught us, 'I came out of the South, and I hope you'll never go back.'"[37]

In Montgomery's Madison Park, where John H. Winston Jr. came of age, his grandparents' advice that he consider becoming a physician owed much to the difficulty of persuading doctors to make house calls in the all-Black neighborhood. As Winston explained: "There were not many Black physicians, or almost none, and when they came out, they came either to pronounce you [dead] or to tell the people you weren't gonna live. Then there were other times when you couldn't get anybody. And as I grew up, I said, 'Well, I'm gonna go into medicine and put all these physicians out of business.'" He recalled the time when his mother became ill and no doctor would visit her: "I was kind of agitated about it. And then [I] became more intense on it. But then, as time went on, I thought that was probably just a dream."[38]

For Winston's cousin, Hagalyn Seay Wilson, becoming a doctor meant more than choosing a profession. "I always felt that I had a mission to fulfill," she said. "I did not know what that mission was in my younger days, but I knew that I was to serve in some area of need. I think I inherited that from my father."[39] After finishing Livingstone College in North Carolina in 1945, Wilson began teaching in Greenville, Alabama, in the same church-related school where her mother had once taught. Later, she took a job in the public schools of Chilton County, north of Montgomery, but soon concluded that the position offered no room for growth.

It was at this point that Wilson remembered the advice of one of her advisors at Livingstone: "He was the dean, and he was from Boston, and he knew of this school in Philadelphia. He knew of Black women who had graduated from the Women's Medical College. He suggested that I become a doctor and that I apply to that school. But it did not occur to me that I wanted to be a doctor. I had never thought about that before."

Wilson applied to the Woman's Medical College, which asked her to come to Philadelphia for an interview. As word got out, she began hearing comments from friends of her family that she would never make it: "I heard from whites and Blacks my parents knew about the money they had spent getting their children ready to go to Harvard for an interview and various other northern schools, and the children had not been accepted. So there was a general feeling that I might not be accepted." Wilson's father neither encouraged nor discouraged her, but it was clear that he thought being a doctor, in her words, was "too much a professional challenge for his daughter" and that he would rather see her marry and have children like her mother.

In the end, Wilson resolved to make her own decision: "That was the first time in my life that I decided, 'Well, if I am going to be accepted, I will have to go. If I'm not going to be accepted, I'll either not go, or they will reject me after I get there.' So I decided that the fifty-dollar round-trip train fare to Philadelphia wasn't too much to try to find out what the answer would be. And from that time until this, I've always decided that I'd never pass up an opportunity to achieve something, that I would just try it and see, especially if I were interested. And that's been my philosophy ever since then."[40] Wilson's decision can be especially appreciated if placed in context. Of the African American doctors practicing in Alabama before 1970, just ten were women, an indication of the obstacles they faced in gaining access to the professions. The problem was not limited to Alabama. Between 1891 and 1940, only sixty-three women received degrees from Howard and fifty-five from Meharry. After World War II, the number started to accelerate, Meharry producing eighty-five and Howard, forty-one from 1960 to 1967 alone.[41]

Women who persevered and were able to gain admission to medical school often had to contend with a dispiriting sexism. Dorothy L. Brown, the South's first Black female surgeon, later recalled the harassment she faced after entering Meharry in 1944 as one of only five women. Most of it came from male students who told her that she should be home raising a family, but in one case, a professor offered to give her an A in his class if she slept with him. The dean casually dismissed Brown's complaint.[42]

Like Wilson, Jefferson Underwood Jr. decided to enter medicine after following the advice of his professors. He had been drafted in 1943 after completing one year at Alabama State and when the war ended was at a loss as to his future. It was not a problem of self-confidence. While in the service, he completed a year of basic engineering courses in the Army Specialized Training Program (ASTP) at West Virginia State and went on to earn the rank of second lieutenant, landing in Europe shortly after D-day. Back in Montgomery, Underwood sought advice from his teachers and from the president of Alabama State: "The majority felt that with my background and studies at West Virginia State, I was quite well-equipped to take a major in premed. So that's when I switched to premed."[43]

Peer influence also influenced the choice of a medical career. By the time he finished Industrial High School in Birmingham, Alexander J. Brewer had decided to become an undertaker, a position of high social rank within the Black community. His thinking changed when he enrolled at Fisk in 1936: "As they were interviewing the students as to what occupation they would pursue, every male was saying medicine. So, I said, 'Hell, I can't be odd. I'll say medicine too.'"[44]

Similarly, Tuskegee surgeon Thomas J. Calhoun had wanted to be a biology teacher, a choice influenced by his admiration for the woman who taught him the subject at the lab school of South Carolina's Claflin College. It was not until his junior year at South Carolina State that he began thinking of medicine: "All the other fellows in my class decided they were going to take the Medical Aptitude Test. So I took it too. And they all decided to apply to med school. So I applied too. Out of my class—this was during the war years—there were six fellows that went to med school. Everybody else was in the army."[45]

For two-thirds of those in our group, the choice of a medical school was fairly straightforward. Meharry led the way, training 62 percent of Alabama's Black doctors before 1970. Next came Howard, with 17.8 percent, and then Leonard, with 8 percent. Assorted Northern and Midwestern schools that had historically admitted a few Black students to each entering class accounted for 12.5 percent. While a few white medical schools in the South began opening their doors to African Americans during the 1950s, it was not until 1965 that the University of Alabama did so.[46]

By 1968, Meharry had produced a national total of 4,522 Black doctors since its founding, as compared with 3,875 for Howard, whose student clientele tended to come from the Northeast and from the states adjoining the District of Columbia. A total of twenty-two in our group received their Howard training during the 1920s and 1930s, the era that saw the opening of the TVAH and the expanding role of Andrew Memorial Hospital. In all, thirteen of our Howard graduates were associated with one or both of these hospitals.

The dominance of Meharry is not surprising. While premed students often applied to both schools to improve their chances of acceptance, the proximity of Meharry to home made it the more appealing choice, despite Howard's better reputation. Alex Carl Hansen, a native of the US Virgin Islands who taught ophthalmology at the school, remembered from his own student days at Meharry during the 1940s that his classmates tended to view Howard as the more prestigious of the two schools, owing to its larger hospital, famous faculty, and federal funding, which spared it the financial stresses suffered by Meharry. On the other hand, Hansen believed that Meharry was equal to Howard academically and that its students were better equipped to do more with less.[47]

Some Black medical students in Alabama after 1948 received modest scholarships resulting from a contract between Meharry and the governors of several Southern and border states. Determined to keep Black people out of their own medical schools, the governors had agreed to provide annual tuition subsidies in the amount of $1,500 for each medical and dental student and $750 for each nursing student from their states. In return, Meharry agreed to reserve a set number of places in each entering class for participating states. Though perpetuating racial segregation in medical education, the arrangement helped to ease the school's financial problems.[48]

LIFE IN MEDICAL SCHOOL

"It was hell trying to get through—first year, second year, third year, fourth year—because I tell you what the story was back in those days: If you flunked, you were out of medicine totally. You didn't go to any other med school in the country, and you couldn't come back to Meharry. You had no second chance."[49] That is how Alexander Lee Brewer described his time at Meharry, where he completed his degree in 1944. He was not alone. Charles E. McGruder, who finished eight years after Brewer, found himself overwhelmed in first-year anatomy:

> It scared the devil out of you when you went into the class and the guy who was handing you a bone said, "Talk to the bone." Every little bump, knot, on the bone has a name, and every little hole of any size is a foramen of something through which passes a nerve or a blood vessel. And of course if you turned this over, looking at the bottom of it, there's a big opening there through which the *medulla oblongata* goes in, and all these nerves and things got different holes they come out of, coming from the brain going out to the body, and that's the kind of thing that would happen. And then *this* process and *that*—the clinoid process, the spinoid process, the foraminal volume, the hiatus of the facial. You were always feeling like, "I've got to work harder to be sure I don't flunk."[50]

During the first year, students were caught up in a whirlwind of written examinations, oral quizzes, demonstrations, and laboratory work. Those who received a failing grade in a course were dropped from Meharry's rolls, and those performing below average, depending on the judgment of the Student Evaluation Committee, were allowed to repeat it only once. J. L. B. Forrester, a Nashville otolaryngologist (an ear, nose, and throat specialist) who received his Meharry degree in 1936 and later taught part time at the school, recalled that seventeen in his class of seventy had flunked out. These rates declined as Meharry became more selective with admissions, though attrition remained high during the freshman year.[51]

At both Meharry and Howard, the first two years focused on the basic sciences, including anatomy, physiology, chemistry, pathology, bacteriology, parasitology, and pharmacology. Dodson M. Curry of Birmingham was stunned by the emphasis on rote learning: "You would say, 'What does this have to do with medicine?' But no one at this stage would tell you. They'd say, 'Learn it, pass this on the examination, or get out.' And certainly, they would weed you out. I mean, it took very few infractions and very few poor grades." Curry never forgot the words of an upperclassman he knew: "It is amazing how much knowledge they can put in your head against your will."[52]

Barefield-Pendleton, who had shown a gift for the sciences in high school and college, found himself drowning the first year. "I think I made ten on my first anatomy test, and I don't mind telling it because I finished the course with an A." He soon discovered his problem—not knowing how to take notes. He also had to overcome the intimidating effects of his peers. In anatomy, for example, there was a student with a master's in psychology and another in math or chemistry: "Another of my classmates—they gave [him] a scholarship for the best record in embryology. This fellow had had the course in college, using the same textbook that we were using in medical school. They were marking on the curve, but the curve didn't mean anything when they set the curve so high."[53]

Montgomery native John H. Winston Jr. shared Barefield-Pendleton's weakness in note-taking, despite having taught a course on the subject while in the Air Force. Medical school, he discovered, required "intense, directed study [where] you covered everything. And when they lectured, they weren't going over it the next day. I was just nonchalantly glancing at it and reading. The tests would come up, and I was making fifty and sixty for the first two or three times. I learned that you have to put more time and intensity on it. [It] was almost Christmas, and by that time I was behind."[54]

Along with anatomy, physiology loomed large the first year. Of those in our group who earned their degrees after 1930, most studied the subject under Daniel T. Rolfe, whose course was required for all medical, dental, and nursing students. A Meharry product who had done postgraduate training at the University of Chicago, he was an imposing figure. Owing to his girth, students secretly referred to him as "The Fat Man," though with a mixture of awe and respect.

The worst times were on Fridays when Rolfe would sit on a stool with his gradebook open on his lap calling out random names. Barefield-Pendleton remembered that he "would give you an examination with three questions. If you missed one, you had sixty-six. And Rolfe had a test every Friday, an oral test, and he would let you talk as long as you wanted, and when you stopped talking, he'd say, 'I'm sorry. I think you missed the point.'"[55] For students who failed a class and were told to leave Meharry, the shock could be severe. Hereford witnessed an example: "Once, I was picking up my grades, and the man in front of me had just gotten his, and still, he didn't move away from the window. Finally, he turned around, and there were tears in his eyes, and he said, 'I'll kill the mother fucker. He's messin' with my *life*.'"[56]

Charles W. Johnson, known for his tough grading standards in bacteriology and parasitology during the 1950s, recalled how his cousin became afraid for Johnson's safety, especially after the latter walked into class one day to see "V-8" written on the blackboard. Someone later explained to him that it referred not to the Ford V8 automobile but to W. E. A. Ford, a Nashville otolaryngologist and part-time faculty member who in the spring of 1939 was shot and killed by a student. His colleague J. L. B. Forrester witnessed the shooting:

Dr. Ford had gotten to class before it started, around ten minutes to eight.

> I got there at about five till eight, and when I got there, Ford saw this guy with a pony [i.e., cheating aid] and immediately took him down to see the president, who said the kid was out. I was trying to explain to Dr. Ford that class hadn't actually started, when the boy comes in with a gun. He pulled open the door and came in and said, "Stay right where you are." And then, pow! pow! pow! I was the only one who saw the killing. He came in and shot him and then ran down that little hall and killed himself. Ford was dead before we could get him to the emergency room.[57]

McGruder recalled that one had no contact with patients during the freshman year and only limited contact during the sophomore year, but "then, during your junior year, you went through all of the disciplines, and you really had to do all the things you're supposed to do as a doctor."[58] Hubbard was Meharry's teaching hospital, and the training there included rotations of four to eight weeks in medicine, surgery, obstetrics, and pediatrics. Clerkships of two students, working in outpatient clinics, gave students the chance to do patient work-ups, including physical examinations, x-rays, and laboratory tests. Most patients were Black, and less than 20 percent could pay the twenty-five-cent registration fee. Alex Carl Hansen remembered that chairs lined the hallways because waiting rooms were full.[59]

Among the most popular teachers was a soft-spoken surgeon named John Henry Hale, known to his colleagues as "Big John," who in 1932 became the first African American to be admitted to the American College of Surgeons. Hansen remembered that he was known among students as the "I Doctor" because of his emphasis on self-esteem and the personal pronoun "I." Hale died in 1944, shortly after Hansen graduated: "In the last part of my senior year, he was in heart failure, and you could see from the beating of his heart through his gown that he had an enlarged heart. And sometimes he would have swelling of his ankles and nosebleed."[60] Barefield-Pendleton saw it too: "He'd be standing up there operating on the patient, and you could look at [Hale's] chest, and you could see his heart just pounding."[61]

Another charismatic professor was Louisiana native Matthew Walker, who was often seen walking the halls of Hubbard Hospital chewing on a big cigar. A graduate of Meharry, where he finished with honors in 1934, Walker did a residency in surgery and gynecology at Hubbard Hospital and later became chair of the Department of Surgery. He followed Hale as the school's dominant figure in the field and often brought surgical residents and senior medical students to the Taborian Hospital in Mound Bayou,

Mississippi, which had been created in 1942 to bring health care to Black people in the Delta.[62]

One of those surgical residents was Walker's own daughter, Charlotte Rose Walker, a Fisk graduate who received her degree at Meharry in 1964 and went on to a distinguished career in cancer surgery. She never forgot her time at Mound Bayou, where she found herself doing mostly primary care: "The people would come, and some of them would be in terrible medical condition. But they were always cooperative, always grateful because they didn't have medical care. They lived in that town on plantations, even though slavery was over. Some of the rich white land owners still owned huge tracts of farmland and ran these places like plantations, and the people were just living there because they couldn't get away."[63]

Calvin R. Dowe found himself at Mound Bayou in 1954 doing a month-long rotating internship, having been "volunteered" for the assignment by Matthew Walker himself. "It wasn't nobody but the two of us," Dowe recalled, "me and McKinley Exum from Memphis, Tennessee. We and another guy named Dr. King, who was a surgical resident, ran the hospital. We were the radiologists. We were the ophthalmologists. We were the obstetricians. And it wasn't no question of could you do it. You just had to do what you could do." What most struck Dowe were the cases of severe hypertension: "I've never seen anybody with blood pressure [so high]. My blood pressure would go up from taking theirs. Sociological people would have to delve into that. All we knew was that it was just so sky high. We would try to tell them to lower their salt intake, but they didn't have any medication."[64]

In obstetrics, Meharry boasted a talented, soft-spoken professor with pince-nez named Walter F. B. James, a native of Georgetown, Guyana, who was known on campus as the "Black Prince" because of his stylish suits and white gloves. Thomas J. Calhoun remembered James's admonitions to his students to develop a light touch in obstetrics, telling them, "You must be elegant." Students liked his teaching but feared his grading standards: "He was a good professor, but he ended a whole lot of fellows' careers too," Calhoun said.[65]

Where abortion was concerned, instruction varied according to the views of the professor, if it was included at all. The neglect is all the more remarkable considering the large numbers of Black women who sought abortions, some because of the hardships an additional child would impose, others because they feared being beaten by their husbands or simply wished to exercise more control over their own bodies.[66] That the obstetrics faculty chose to be cautious is understandable. In Tennessee, as in Alabama, abortion was illegal before 1973 and carried the possibility of fines and imprisonment. The only exceptions allowed by law were those in which childbirth posed a threat to the mother's health (rape and incest exceptions were added in the late 1960s).

Throughout the 1940s and 1950s, the Nashville press regularly depicted crackdowns on abortionist "rings" in the city, which often consisted of an elderly Black woman or a Meharry graduate long since retired. Recognizing the damage that a Black doctor could suffer if he or she became known as a "physician-abortionist," one Meharry professor urged that, once in practice, students reject such requests within earshot of their waiting rooms. Edgar Bass Keemer Jr., who claimed to have done over thirty thousand abortions during his years of practice in Detroit, recalled that abortion techniques were not taught at all while he was at Meharry during the 1930s.[67]

Whether the harsh pedagogical techniques employed at Meharry produced the best results can only be guessed at. By contrast, the atmosphere at Howard seems to have been more sympathetic toward students. James T. Montgomery had warm memories of his years at Howard, whose faculty impressed him with their empathy and teaching ability. He especially admired his anatomy professor, Montague Cobb, who had trained in both medicine and anthropology: "He was concerned about Black students in general. He spent a lot of the time, I remember, trying to prove that there was no difference between Black and white folks."[68]

Howard enrolled a half dozen or so white medical students each year, one of whom Montgomery met soon after arriving on campus. The entering class had just assembled on the steps of a building to have its freshmen picture taken when one of the white students came over and started a conversation. Montgomery recalled his words: "He said, 'I want to tell you something. I may not be number one in this class when it finishes, but the person who's number one will know I will be breathing down his neck.' And to my mind, he said that because he looked around, and all the folks were Black except four or five of them, and he thought there were only four or five people to compete with. And I said to myself, 'I don't know where you're going to finish, but you're going to finish somewhere behind me.' And he finished miles behind me. I was lucky enough to be the top honors student in my class at Howard in 1953."[69]

At Woman's Medical College of Pennsylvania, which she entered in 1950, Montgomery's Hagalyn Seay Wilson found an acceptance that she had rarely known in an integrated setting, far different from what Selma's Pauline E. Dinkins experienced back in 1919. In a letter that Dinkins wrote to the dean of the Woman's Medical College after returning to practice in Selma, she made no attempt to hide her feelings: "I was never able to make myself feel like a real member of the class, nor even like a part of the college. I surely tried to do this, but I failed. Every bit of my energy was taken in forcing myself to stay to the end. You see, it simply infuriates me to hear one ill word said about the negro race. The first occasions of unhappiness on my part arose in the first week of my junior year when a colored woman with arthritis was presented in surgery clinical conference. The clinician said, 'Because of her race,' etc. From that day, I was truly sensitive beyond measure. And never did I recover from one wound before I received another." [70]

Things had changed by the time Wilson arrived. Though she was one of only three Black students among two hundred, she thought it was far better than being at Meharry, where she was also accepted. "I had a cousin who was at Meharry," she later said, "and he told me of the unpleasant experiences that the females had in the medical school with the males there." Not that there were no moments of doubt: "During my freshman year, I was really frightened because most of the other girls in my class were from the Big Ten universities and from the Ivy League schools, and I was from Alabama. And I could remember those classes [in Alabama] where we never passed the middle of the book, never knew what was in the last half of the book."

Wilson's salvation was a neuroanatomist named Hartwick Kuhlenbeck, who stopped her one day in the hall between classes to ask if she was having any trouble with bone quizzes: "And I just felt like he was rooting for me, because Dr. Kuhlenbeck was not a person to stop and talk with anybody. He encouraged me more than anybody else just by stopping and offering me assistance if I needed any. That helped me get through the first year because it helped me to develop the confidence that I needed."[71]

LICENSURE EXAMINATIONS AND INTERNSHIPS

During the early years of the century, Black medical graduates had performed poorly on state licensure examinations. Those from Howard tended to do better than those from Meharry and Leonard, its failure rate, based on a sampling of twelve states, standing at 24.3 percent in 1906. That compared with an astonishing 45.9 percent failure rate for Meharry and 42.8 for Leonard. In an effort to explain these showings, Meharry president George W. Hubbard cited racial discrimination on the part of white examiners but was quick to add other factors as well—namely, the absence of intellectual stimulation in the student's early life, the weakness of literary and scientific education in the Black schools, and poverty, which compelled many medical students to work while attending school.[72]

For all Black doctors practicing in Alabama before 1970, approximately 70 percent passed state boards. Most took their examinations in Alabama (56.7 percent), though others did so in neighboring states like Tennessee (17 percent) and Georgia (7 percent) under a system known as reciprocity. A sampling of seventy-six examination scores from the Alabama group shows a wide range of performances. Averaging the numerical scores that examiners assigned to each of the ten sections of the test reveals that forty candidates (53 percent) scored eighty or higher, including four in the nineties. On their initial attempt, seven scored below the minimum seventy-five needed for a pass.

By the 1920s, the failure rate of Meharry graduates on state boards across the country had fallen to 26 percent, and with implementation of more rigorous admissions standards and the hiring of better faculty, the figure by 1930 had dropped to just over 12 percent. In 1946, it stood at 7 percent, still higher than the failure rate for graduates of white medical schools, but lower than the 9.9 percent for candidates from all approved medical schools in the United States and abroad.[73]

For the earliest graduates in our group, there was little need to ponder the choice of internships because few were available. Biographical data for 105 of the 125 who completed their degrees in 1920 or earlier contain no mention of their having done a fifth year of training. In fact, Alabama was one of twenty-five states that did not require an internship in order to receive a medical license. In 1935, Henry Arthur Callis, professor of medicine at Howard, noted that while most graduates of Howard and Meharry at that time did internships, around 40 percent of Black doctors who were currently in practice in the United States had not been able to do so.[74] By that point, the possibilities for hospital training started to improve. Of 119 African Americans who graduated from medical school in 1927, a total of seventy-one were able to do internships, and by 1939, the number had risen to 168. M. O. Bousfield, director of the Negro Health Division of the Julius Rosenwald Fund, noted that for Black doctors "the internship is no longer an optional choice."[75]

Even then, African American doctors were largely confined to fourteen Black hospitals approved by the AMA and the American College of Surgeons. Citing figures for 1932, Numa P. G. Adams, dean of the School of Medicine at Howard, pointed out that for 4,814 white medical graduates, there were 6,044 internships available; for 122 Black medical graduates, there were only 110, all of them confined to the fourteen approved hospitals. Only with the civil rights movement did this straitjacket begin to loosen. By 1969, the combined 137 graduates of Howard and Meharry were interning at sixty-four hospitals across the nation. By 1972, the number had risen to eighty-eight—thirty-seven from Howard and fifty-one from Meharry.[76]

Among Alabama's doctors, the heaviest concentrations for internships were at City Hospital No. 2 in St. Louis and its successor, Homer G. Phillips; Freedmen's Hospital in Washington, DC; and Hubbard Hospital in Nashville. Smaller numbers trained at Harlem Hospital, Andrew Memorial, Kansas City General No. 2, and, starting in the 1950s, assorted Catholic hospitals serving large numbers of indigent Black people.

Overshadowing all others was Homer G. Phillips. Built in a Black business and residential district of North St. Louis and dedicated in 1937, the massive art deco structure had 685 beds and was one of the largest hospitals in the country. The city's stinginess in funding its operations, however, often led to shortages of staff, which helps explain why Calvin R. Dowe felt overwhelmed on his first day: "My first rotation was to medicine. They took me and showed me where the ward was, and that was my orientation. You learned in that situation to do what you could. If you would just look at it, you'd say it was impossible. It's so many sick people. They're all poor people, don't have nothin'. The first day I had to go to the pediatric clinic, I just knew I couldn't. I said, 'They gotta be kidding.' You don't see all these people. But after a couple of weeks, you'd see all them people and take care of 'em and get 'em on out of there." [77]

James T. Montgomery, who had come to Homer G. Phillips a year before Dowe arrived, was likewise unimpressed by the quality of instruction but determined to use the hospital's resources to advance his knowledge. "Homer G. Phillips was a place where you could learn," he said. "You had the experience of seeing every type of disease that mankind could have. The teaching program wasn't worth anything; you always had to teach yourself." [78] After completing his internship, Montgomery decided to stay on for a three-year residency in internal medicine, which allowed him to learn from those professors at nearby Washington University School of Medicine who supervised the residents' training. In addition, Homer G. Phillips granted him a one-year leave to go to Harvard to study with noted cardiologist Louis Wolff.

As he approached the end of his residency, Montgomery began receiving inquiries from medical practices in Kansas City and Toledo regarding their interest in his joining them. He turned them down, determined to return to Birmingham. "It was home, that was number one," he said, "and number two, in 1950, while doing my first year [at Howard], I had married a young lady from Birmingham named Althea Palmer, and we'd been married for seven years. And because of that, I knew I was coming back to Birmingham." Montgomery was under no illusions as to what awaited him on his return: "Everybody understood that it was separate and totally unequal. If you were Black, your life in the courts still wasn't worth very much. You knew to get in your separate line, and you didn't feel so bad being there, though you knew it wasn't right, because you'd accept a lot of things in those days."[79]

Montgomery's thinking mirrored that of many other Black graduates from Alabama. After finishing Meharry in 1951, Maynard V. Foster became the first Black intern appointed to the staff of Hurley Medical Center in Flint, Michigan. His wife, Alma W. Foster, recalled how his superior performance in the job resulted in several offers that would have enabled him to remain in Flint. "It was very tempting," she said, "and he had almost made up his mind to stay there, and he later made a trip home, and he saw such a need that he just decided that he'd go back [to Mobile]."[80] Dodson M. Curry never had any doubts: "I had my parents here. I knew the lay of the land, the whole philosophy, and how to avoid pitfalls and all of these kinds of things, where[as] in other cities it was six on one hand and a half dozen on the other. When it came down to practical things, this is the way it was. There was never any question whether I would come back here."[81]

John H. Winston Jr., who had interned at St. Margaret's Hospital in Hammond, Indiana, and completed a residency in general surgery at the TVAH, remembered that "it was my intention to come back here all the time. I had no reason not to come because my parents were here, most of my relatives were here, and I could walk into a situation, and I'd have enough relatives to treat to make a living." Hagalyn Seay Wilson put it more succinctly: "It never occurred to me to do anything but return to Alabama."[82]

REGION OF PRACTICE

Figure 2.2 shows the location by county and region for the 241 licensed Black physicians practicing in Alabama before 1970. In all, Black doctors were present in twenty-seven of the state's sixty-seven counties.

Although forty-four doctors moved their practices inside the state at some point, a breakdown of the regions where the 241 spent the bulk of their careers shows significant patterns.[83] For example, the heaviest concentrations were in the Black Belt, which accounted for eighty doctors (33 percent) and whose Black population in 1940 numbered 366,000. This included Tuskegee, where thirty-one doctors were located. As we have seen, additional numbers

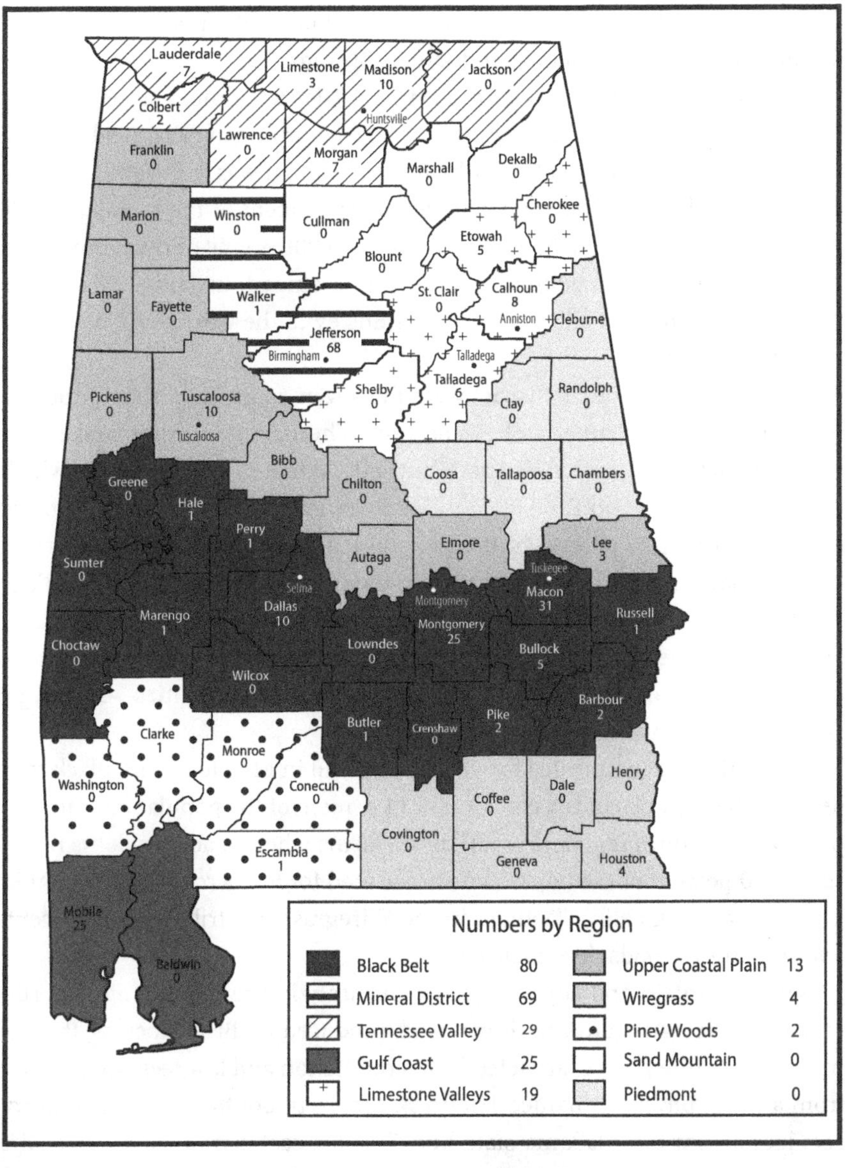

Map 2.2. Distribution of Black physicians by county and region in Alabama, 1879–1970

of Black specialists worked as full-time government employees at the TVAH but, for purposes of comparison, were included in the database only if they had part-time practices on the side. Outside Tuskegee, the proportion of Black doctors in the Black Belt falls to just under 20 percent, of which most were found in Montgomery, Selma, and Union Springs.

Next, with 28.6 percent, was the Mineral District, almost all of its Black doctors being located in Birmingham or its coal-producing and steel-making suburbs. In Jefferson County, of which Birmingham was the seat, Black people numbered over 179,000 in 1940, about 38 percent of the population. By the 1950s, their numbers had risen to over 200,000, many of them employed in the iron and coal industries and living in cramped, unsanitary dwellings in North Birmingham and Southside, in Ensley to the west and Titusville to the southwest.[84]

Following the Mineral District were the seven counties of the Tennessee Valley in North Alabama, with 12 percent. There, cotton farms and textile mills characterized such cities as Huntsville, Athens, and Florence, which usually had one or two Black doctors each. In 1940, Black residents of these counties formed 26 percent of their combined populations, with the largest towns usually containing between seven thousand and eight thousand Black residents. Roughly the same patterns applied to the Limestone Valleys, an area that included the cotton plantations of the Coosa River Valley and produced 7.8 percent of our doctors, all of them in just three cities—Talladega, Gadsden, and Anniston.

The Gulf Coast accounted for 10.3 percent, all in Mobile, where Black residents in the city and county constituted 34 percent of the population. The Upper Coastal Plain, a region of small cotton farms where Black residents represented 30 percent of the population, accounted for 5.3 percent, all of them in Tuscaloosa and Opelika. Dothan, in the Wiregrass, contributed 1.6 percent, and the Piney Woods, less than 1 percent.

Sand Mountain and adjacent Jackson County in the mountainous northeast, where few African Americans lived, produced no Black doctors, though many poor white people, attracted by his reputation and low fees, sought care from a Black physician named Hiram B. Moore in South Pittsburg, Tennessee, just across the Alabama state line. The six east-central counties of the Piedmont produced no Black doctors, though African Americans made up 30 percent of the population. The area's small towns and crossroads and an exploitative system of share cropping were hardly tempting to Black medical graduates. Conditions there are illustrated in Theodore Rosengarten's *All*

God's Dangers, the oral history of a Black sharecropper in Tallapoosa County named Ned Cobb and his fight for social justice during the Depression.[85]

These figures do not reflect how changes over time affected the availability of Black doctors for African Americans. Helpful in this regard are the data published in 1945 by Howard bacteriologist Paul B. Cornely that are based on a study of 144 cities in both North and South, which allow us to compare the medical ratios of our doctors with those of similarly sized cities. Cornely discovered that Black people living in Alabama's largest cities had far less access to Black doctors than those in the nation as a whole, where cities of over fifty thousand averaged one Black doctor per 1,983 African Americans. Both Montgomery and Mobile, for example, were at the bottom when compared to cities of comparable size, the ratio of Black physicians in the former being one per 4,319 Black people and in the latter, one per 4,149. Birmingham itself saw its Black medical corps decline to just nineteen individuals, which produced a ratio of one Black doctor per 5,734 African Americans. Figure 2.3 is based on Cornely's figures.

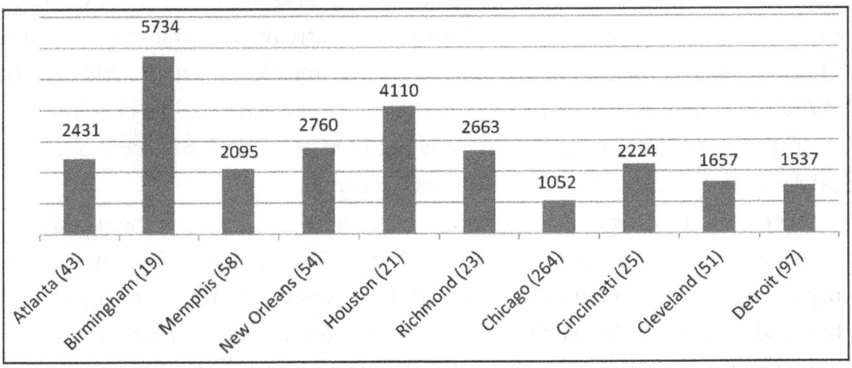

Figure 2.3. Black population per Black physician in Birmingham and in selected cities having over fifty thousand African Americans, 1942. (Numbers derived from Paul B. Cornely, "Distribution of Negro Physicians in the United States in 1942," *Journal of the American Medical Association* 124 [May 1944]: 826–30.)

The poor showing for Birmingham, which had once attracted significant numbers of Black doctors, tells a painful story of bigotry and denial of opportunity. In a reversal of the idealism that had brought many medical graduates back to their home state during the early years of the twentieth century, increasing numbers by the 1930s and 1940s were leaving the city. Four years after Cornely's report, Lionel F. Swan, president of the Mineral District Medical Society, and Ransey G. Cole, its secretary, described in the *Birmingham*

News how desperate conditions had become: "Consider these facts: There are in this area 24 Negro physicians. Of this number, one is away for study. One is temporarily retired because of illness; three others are doing very limited work for the same reason; five are over 60 years of age; and three are reported to be making active plans to move their practices elsewhere. This means that unless new men come into the field, we shall have in this area in five years, about one dozen Negro physicians to care for the needs of 210,000 Negroes."[86]

Our study will now shift its focus to the experiences of Alabama's Black doctors once in practice. No matter how good their training, their professional lives were circumscribed by two powerful realities: The first was the discrimination they faced at the hands of the white medical establishment. The second was the magnitude of health problems within the African American community.

In Alabama, as across the nation, morbidity and mortality rates were highest among Black people, including tuberculosis, heart disease, hypertension, stroke, pulmonary disorders, pneumonia, influenza, and kidney disease. Black death rates, which in 1950 stood at 11.4 per thousand residents (as opposed to 8.2 for white people), reflected an endless stream of personal tragedies. "Things like breast cancer we saw very late," recalled John H. Winston Jr. "We'd see a lot of cancer of the uterus that was far advanced, lots of colon cancer that'd been far advanced. That was because of the lack of access to medical care, and sometimes it might be other things."[87]

Lack of education and ignorance of preventive care were twin realities that both Black and white doctors confronted on a daily basis. Compounding these for African American practitioners was their exclusion from white hospitals and such life-saving resources as were available there. While our doctors were sometimes called upon to repair the effects of harmful folk practices—ashes and soot packed into an open wound, for example, or fatty meat and goose grease applied to an abscess—the oral histories show that large numbers of African Americans, far from rejecting scientific medicine, openly embraced it.

CHAPTER THREE

Physicians to the Poor

Once in practice, Alabama's Black physicians had to adjust their financial expectations to the poverty of their patients. That meant accepting partial payments for their services or, as was often the case, no payments at all. The doctors' exclusion from the hospitals further depressed their earnings, as did the distrust they often encountered among the Black middle classes. "You will find that the only people who are going to support you are the poorest people," Birmingham's Black surgeon Hampton Brewer once remarked. "It is not the well-to-do or middle class Black that will support a Black doctor but the poorest on the totem pole."[1]

This chapter will show how Black physicians tried with only limited success to establish a footing in Alabama during the Jim Crow era. In the process—and contrary to what they would have wished had they enjoyed a system that rewarded their talents—they provided at least sporadic sources of health care for the poorest African Americans. The oral accounts presented here show how members of our group sought to cope with low fees and nonpayment for services by increasing the numbers of patients they treated. At the same time, these numbers bore witness to the desire of many poor African Americans to be treated by Black doctors.

GETTING STARTED

African American practitioners generally worked in professional isolation, sometimes in offices attached to their homes or in small clinics located in Black neighborhoods. Those who practiced in large towns and cities often had offices in the Black business districts or in buildings owned by fraternal orders, such as the eight-story Masonic Temple Building in Birmingham. While their material circumstances differed greatly, graduates of Meharry and Howard usually needed money to get their practices up and running, but that was not always easy.

On leaving the army after his service in Korea, Barefield-Pendleton practiced in Mobile for a year before deciding to go elsewhere: "I didn't do too well financially in Mobile 'cause five of us came in at the same time, five new physicians, Black. So I was slow getting off the ground. And I said, 'You know, this just doesn't make sense. I got a wife and two children, and I know I can do better than this somewhere else.'" A drug representative suggested that he consider the unincorporated Black community in southwest Birmingham known as Roosevelt City. It was a poor district, but it gave him access to Black industrial workers in nearby Bessemer.

In seeking a loan to pay for his moving expenses, Barefield-Pendleton assumed that his existing practice would put him in good stead. Instead, he had to take out a loan on his car just to get his possessions off the van. That was only the start, as became evident when the drug representative took him down to a bank to get an investment loan: "They wouldn't okay it. He was pretty sure he could get a loan for me because he had knowledge of white physicians who came in the same time I came in, and he said they didn't have a loan problem of $10,000."[2]

In Montgomery, Jefferson Underwood Jr. had better luck after asking a local bank for a loan of $5,000. The bank president said that he would first have to check the doctor's record at the University at Buffalo; a few days later, he called to report that he had spoken with several of Underwood's professors who said that if he failed to repay the loan, they would do so themselves. In the meantime, Martin Luther King Jr., who had become pastor of Dexter Avenue Baptist Church and Underwood's patient, cheered him on: "I went into practice in '56, but I was here part of '55 as well. I knew Rev. King before the bus boycott, before he became so famous, and we became pretty close. After I set up practice and the bus boycott began, I was active in the civil rights movement, and King just told people, 'We got this doctor in town. Go to him!'"[3]

Also providing encouragement and advice was the venerable Roman T. Adair, whom Underwood had idolized since childhood. During summer breaks from medical school, he would often stop by the aging doctor's house for a visit, sometimes driving him on his house calls after his eyes began failing him. Adair had been a formidable presence in the Black community since opening a practice on Monroe Street in 1911. He had served on the Board of

Trustees of Hale Infirmary, organized the all-Black Capital City Medical Society, and, during the Depression, had led the drive to create a Montgomery branch of the Negro Civic Improvement League. Adair was reputed to be one of the wealthiest African Americans in the city, though he spent much of his time caring for the indigent sick. In her autobiography, children's author Ellen Tarry recounted a tour of the City of St. Jude during the early 1950s, where she found Dr. Adair, assisted by one of the sisters, treating the sick and performing minor operations.[4]

Three years later, Adair's life spiraled downward after he shot and killed his wife of thirty-nine years on suspicion of adultery. Released on a $10,000 bond, he was eventually acquitted by a sympathetic jury, possibly owing to his advanced age and his earlier services to the community, but could not escape a blistering public humiliation at the hands of Rev. Vernon Johns, the blunt-speaking predecessor of Martin Luther King, Jr. at Dexter Avenue Baptist Church.[5]

Like Adair, Underwood opened his office in a large upstairs space on Monroe Street, which he partitioned off to create a waiting room, an x-ray room, a consultation room, and three small examining rooms. He remembered Monroe Street as being "*the* street" where most of the city's Black physicians were located and where Black people from the city and county poured in every Saturday: "They could get rides to come to town. This was their one-note shopping centers. You bought your groceries there. You went to the movies there."[6]

Things did not at first go so smoothly for John H. Winston Jr. Along with his partner, Julius Pryor Jr., a fellow of the American Board of Surgery who had degrees in both medicine and dentistry, Winston had envisioned a surgery center that could serve Black people in Montgomery County and surrounding areas. Having decided to build rather than to rent, the two found a lot for sale on Oak Street, not far from St. Jude Hospital. Despite their credentials, a local bank refused them a loan, and they ended up borrowing from Puritan Life and Health and the Small Business Bureau. In the end, it all worked out: "We had the office, we had the waiting room, we had the library, we had a laboratory. [Pryor] was a dentist also; so we had one dental room we called the ENT [ear, nose, and throat] room. We had about three or four examining rooms and a big waiting room. We started out with one nurse, and my wife was the secretary. His wife was the lab technician, and then we added a number of more rooms because over the years we sometimes had four or five other doctors in there. We've had several people rotate through."[7] Hagalyn Seay Wilson, who in 1957 became the first Black woman to practice in

Montgomery, chose to ignore the banks altogether, instead using the AS Aloe Company, a St. Louis firm that sold medical supplies and that, in her words, "set up doctors all over the United States for fifty dollars down and literally a hundred dollars a month." Even then, things were difficult: "I think it was harder for a female. Most of the males who preceded me had professional wives, and the wives had jobs, and I would say I didn't think that they had as hard a time as I. The only difference is they usually came when someone else was leaving, and so many of them sort of inherited practices. I didn't inherit a practice when I came here."[8]

Like Underwood, Wilson rented space on Monroe Street, but the location left her uneasy: "I was a little fearful because even at that time, the people who decided to enjoy themselves on the weekends were the people who frequented Monroe Street, and at any time I was afraid that I would look up and see someone coming at me with the victim of a stab wound, because hospitalization was not readily available at the time, and the doctors performed a lot of services in their offices that they wouldn't think of performing at this time. So I was a little afraid of Monroe Street."

Offering constant encouragement was again Dr. Adair, who had an office next door. Wilson remembered him as being "very articulate, very immaculate in his dress. He wore gloves that I believe were white suede gloves on his hands all the time. He went to Harvard every summer for refresher courses. He was just the cream of the crop." She was grateful for Adair's many tips: "He told me about all the things to expect. He told me about the Easter snap—the people would be in town to buy Easter outfits for their children, and they would not have money for the doctor. He told me about the Christmas snap and all the little things that you couldn't learn in medical school."

Three years into her practice, Wilson purchased property on Jeff Davis Avenue in the city's heavily Black west side, using funds she had saved by putting aside five to ten dollars a week: "We had patients all day at three dollars—it may have been five dollars by then, but it was three dollars when I first came here. I lived in apartments in the back of my office for the first ten years. That saved a little money, but you might also get a knock on your door at any time night or day."[9]

In Birmingham, Dodson M. Curry was able to reestablish himself in the same office he had vacated after being drafted and sent to Korea as a combat medic. It was located on 7th Avenue North in a house previously occupied by an elderly Black physician named Edward H. Ballard (the house would later be owned by the Black surgeon Herschell Lee Hamilton, who treated injured civil rights workers there during the 1960s). As best as Curry could recall, Ballard, who had served the Black community since the early 1930s, had gotten into trouble with the authorities regarding his obstetrical practices and left for California in order to pursue a career in real estate.

The trouble to which Curry referred involved Dr. Ballard's conviction in the spring of 1950, followed by a suspended sentence of 180 days, for signing birth certificates when he was not present for the deliveries. Instead, the deliveries had been performed by his employee Ida May Wright, a registered Black nurse who was convicted of practicing as a midwife without a license. In his defense, Ballard noted that there were only twenty Black physicians to attend Jefferson County's 175,000 Black residents, a point made also by his attorney, the Black lawyer Arthur Shores, who pointed out that few white physicians would enter the homes of expectant Black mothers to deliver babies. At a farewell banquet for Ballard in August, leaders of the Greater Birmingham Negro Business League and the Mineral District Medical Society expressed their indignation at what they considered the racially biased decision of the court.[10]

Ballard had wanted Curry to buy the practice, but Curry declined, saying that he wished to start his own. Subsequently, the house was sold, and Curry rented the office space. In his words, "I got the practice, the records, and everything there, including the equipment, but I later replaced the equipment. I just walked in and started practicing." Curry's office was fairly typical of Black practices in the city—a large waiting room with benches along the walls, a small consultation room, an examination room, and a physio-therapy room: "You had scales, an examination table, a pediatrics table, two instrument cabinets, and a little linen cabinet."[11]

James T. Montgomery's startup also proved to be easy, mainly because he had saved $4,000 by working in the offices of several St. Louis doctors during his residency, though it was against the rules. As in Curry's case, Montgomery was able to take over the office of a Black physician named Louis D. Green, who had decided to move his practice to Cleveland. With his wife, Electa Green, a Meharry-trained dentist, Green had transformed a modest building in North Birmingham into a small medical center with an x-ray machine, to which Montgomery added an EKG machine he had purchased while finishing his studies at Harvard: "[Green] had a little laboratory back there—you could do CBCs [complete blood count], your analyses, some basic lab work. And it was the nicest office in town."[12]

The problem was that Green's clinic was in a high-crime area. "I had a very good friend who said, 'No, don't go to North Birmingham. That's not a place for you to go,' Montgomery said. "But after looking at the buildings, I drove through ACIPCO [American Cast Iron Pipe Company], which is on the western side of North Birmingham, and I drove through Cottageville, which is the northwestern side of North Birmingham, and I said, 'All these folks out here, I know I can build up a practice.'" While moving into Green's building, Montgomery made a lucky find: It was thirteen hundred cards containing the names and addresses of Green's patients. Montgomery decided to forego the usual practice of visiting Black churches to announce his arrival; instead, he and his wife sat at the dining room table of her grandparents' house during the summer of 1957, addressing envelopes to all those listed on the cards and notifying them of the new practice.[13]

In contrast to his big-city colleagues, Hiram B. Moore had little money saved after he finished his internship and returned to South Pittsburg in 1944. During the first few weeks, he practiced out of his car: "I didn't have an office, didn't have a telephone, but people were sending to get me." He had a telephone put in at his cousin Nora's house, where he was living, but continued "doctoring out of the car" while making house calls. He was finally able to rent space above the meeting hall of the Knights of Pythias, a Black fraternal order. Following a fire there shortly afterward, the president of Lodge Manufacturing, famed for its cast-iron cookware and eager to help out a Black doctor willing to treat the town's workers for low fees, told him to make a call on the president of the local bank, which owned property in a coal yard.

As a result, Moore was able to purchase half the lot at a good price. The president of another industry, Stove Foundry, helped him build an office on the site: "There was no running water. That was during the war, and pipes were hard to get hold of. And [I had] one of them coal stoves. The house was wired for 120 [volts], and I could have got an electric stove, but it had to be 220. I couldn't get the man to rewire it on a 220, and we just done without."[14]

For equipment, Moore started out with a diathermy machine, which produced deep heat for treating muscles and joints, and a cautery, which was used to seal blood vessels in order to prevent bleeding. Sulfa drugs were in use when he started his practice in 1944, and penicillin came on the market in June of the following year. In fact, he was the first doctor in town to use penicillin, having acquired a supply from the hospital where he had interned in North Carolina.

Because patients needing an x-ray or an electrocardiogram had to go to Chattanooga, Moore resolved to learn these procedures himself. Accordingly, in 1952 he took a short course at Cook County Graduate School of Medicine in Chicago and then at New York University School of Medicine, where he learned how to read x-rays and electrocardiograms. "I came back and bought [an EKG machine]," he later recalled. "I [was] the only doctor around here who could read them." Even with his additional training, Moore knew the limitations of his knowledge: "I didn't learn all that technical stuff. I learned how to tell if one was normal. If something was wrong and I couldn't figure it out, *then* I'd send them [to Chattanooga]."[15]

When he began his practice, Moore made sure to pay courtesy calls on the local white doctors, knowing full well how hostility from one or more could damage his prospects. He had not forgotten what a white doctor had told one of Moore's Black colleagues in a neighboring town: "We won't do anything to run you away, but we can make your people run you away." Moore explained that this was accomplished by petty slander: "The Black people were domestics. They're working in the kitchen and all that. So all [the white doctor] has got to do is just drop it one or two times about the Black doctor, and it gets all over the Black community."[16]

RELATIONS WITH WHITE PRACTITIONERS

At its best—and even when racial norms were strictly observed—the relationship of Black doctors with their white colleagues was tenuous, complicated by the degree to which the former had to rely on the latter. Engaged mainly in primary care and with few specialists of their own, Black doctors had to be able to consult with white surgeons and obstetricians in difficult cases and to maintain friendly connections with those willing to admit their patients to the segregated wards of white hospitals. Some white doctors understood the situation. The oral histories mention numerous individuals who were willing to help out Black colleagues, though this had its limits. While encouraging, or at least tolerating, the presence of Black physicians in a community, there were always those, as Hereford observed, who would say things "to let you know they didn't appreciate your pointing poor people in their direction."[17]

Where paying Black patients were concerned, competition played a direct role, a pattern that reflected the distribution of doctors across the state. While there was one white practitioner per 1,732 inhabitants of both races in Alabama as a whole in 1950, more than half were concentrated in Birmingham, Mobile, Montgomery, Huntsville, and Tuscaloosa. Figure 3.1 shows where the state's 1,768 white physicians were located in 1950.

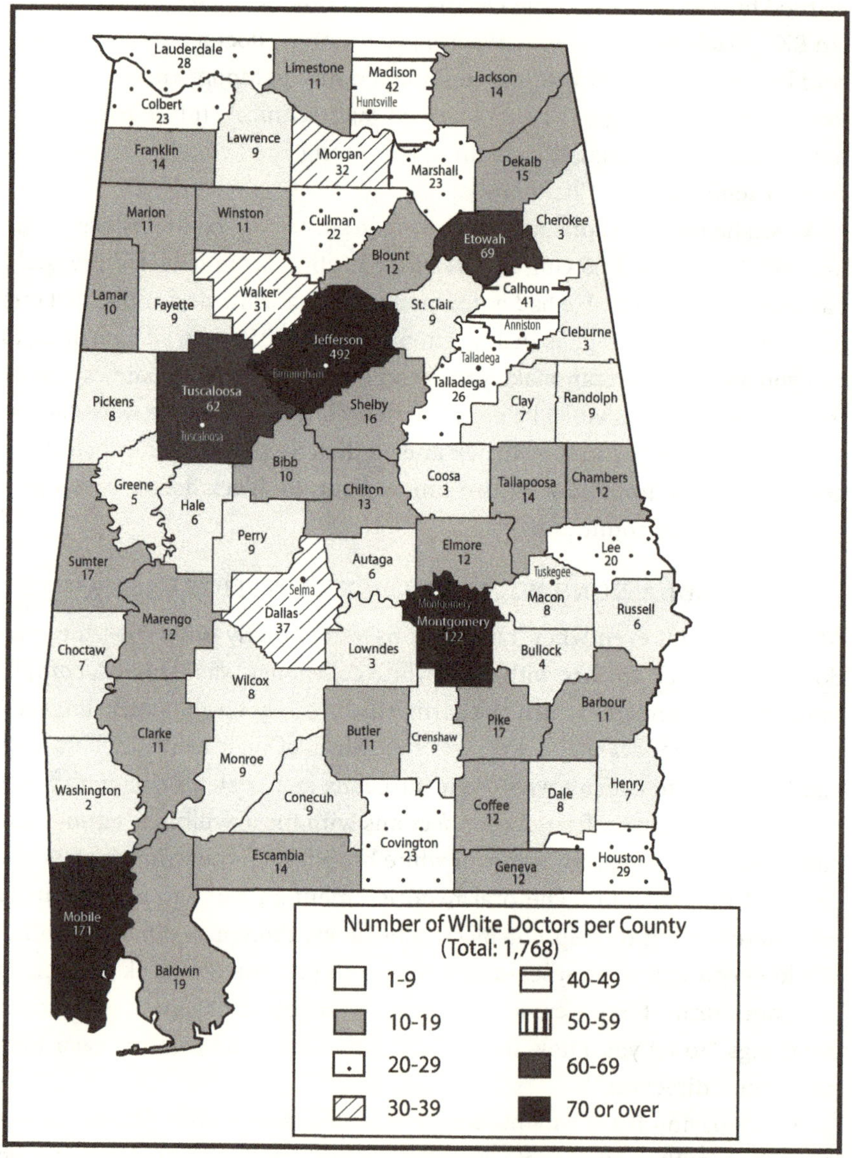

Map 3.1 Distribution of white physicians in Alabama, 1950

Black physicians, too, sought out locations having the best prospects, which excluded large swaths of rural Alabama. There, money was scarce, illiteracy high, and a medical culture nonexistent. In 1969, Carter L. Marshall, a professor in the Department of Community Health at the Mount Sinai School of Medicine in New York, spent six days investigating conditions in the Black Belt's Greene County. He was struck by the ways in which racism affected health services in the region, where Eutaw, the county seat, with a population of 2,700, was the only incorporated town, and where white residents, though outnumbered by Black residents four to one, owned all the businesses and 75 percent of the land.

Marshall noted that despite the existence of a new hospital in Eutaw, most Black residents knew little about its services and, in any case, could not afford its average cost of twenty-six dollars a day. Moreover, the four white physicians in town maintained segregated waiting rooms, which Black patients resented. There had been talk of recruiting a Black physician, but, Marshall said, even if one could be persuaded to come to Greene County, he could not hope to borrow money to open an office, assuming that any white people would sell him land.[18]

The absence of African American doctors in Alabama's rural areas is reflected in the overall ratios of practitioners to population, which show only marginal improvement over time. In 1910, there was one Black doctor per 14,192, which by 1970 had decreased to one per 11,887. Figure 3.2 provides a comparative look at the numbers.

Large towns and cities thus offered Black doctors the best hopes for getting ahead. In Birmingham in 1950, fourteen of the city's twenty-five Black physicians had their offices in the industrial districts of Bessemer, Fairfield, Ensley, and North Birmingham, where steady paychecks, however low in comparison to those of white workers, improved the chances of getting paid. That idea was on Barefield-Pendleton's mind when he started off in Pascagoula: "At that time, there was a shipyard, and this was the type of thing I was interested in. I was reared on a farm, and I knew that money came in once a year. That was in the fall when they harvest the crops, and I didn't particularly like that type of thing."[19]

Without question, some white doctors treated Black patients with dignity and compassion. Ophelia Burnett Northcross remembered from her childhood in Mobile during the 1930s that an elderly white physician named Leon V. McVay, though maintaining a segregated waiting room, was "a god to the Black community," always willing to make house calls and charging just two

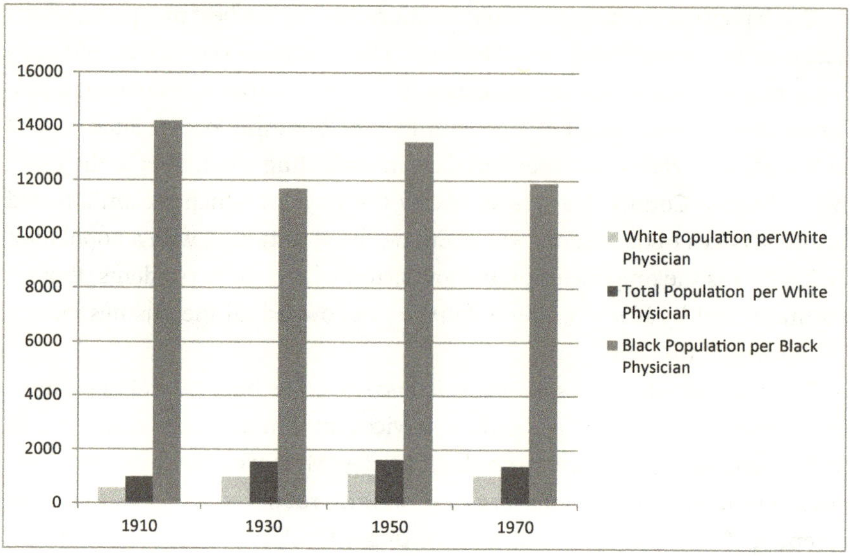

Figure 3.2. Race and medical ratios in Alabama, 1910–1970

dollars a visit.[20] In rural Lawrence County, ninety-four-year-old Hattie Swope had good memories of the white doctors who had treated her: "Mostly would be white doctors when [Black people] would have a family doctor. After I married, [Dr.] Hall would come from Moulton up there. He's the one that said he [wanted to] send me over to a bone doctor in Decatur. He say something's wrong with my bones. It wasn't my bones. It was fluid. The bone doctor examined me, and it wasn't nothin' in my bones. It was high blood [pressure] and fluid. So that doctor sent me to [a white doctor named] Wiley, what's dead. This Wiley treat me nice."[21]

Nevertheless, a Black person who visited a white doctor had to endure a variety of indignities, starting with segregated waiting areas, where one might sit for hours in a cramped room or on a porch. Once admitted into the examining room, patients were typically addressed by white physicians by their first names, a practice that pervaded all levels of medical care. William A. Kates Jr., a New Jersey native who in 1949 began practicing in the town of Madison, west of Huntsville, later recalled from his first days on the job writing a prescription for a Black woman who took it downstairs to the pharmacist: "He called me on the phone and said, 'We don't have any Mrs. So-and-So in town. Who did you write that for?' I said, 'That Black lady who was just up here.' He said, 'Oh, you mean Lizzie,' or whoever it was. 'We don't call them Mr. or Mrs.'"[22]

The paternalism that marked a Black person's dealings with white doctors posed several dangers, not the least of which was the latter's tendency to provide only cursory examinations or to regard patient complaints with less seriousness than they merited. When Dr. Montgomery began practicing in Birmingham in 1957, he found that most of his patients who had been seeing white doctors had never had a physical examination. Elderly women, he recalled, would sometimes say, "I ain't ever had nobody looking under my clothes but my husband."[23]

Lacking specialists of their own, Black physicians were compelled to maintain ties with a few sympathetic members of the county medical society, sometimes assisting them in operations performed on the Black doctor's patients. Such activities often placed Black practitioners in a delicate situation, facing the pain of being rebuffed by white nurses or other members of the hospital staff, eager to remind them that their medical degrees did not confer equality. The same pattern applied to the Black doctor's interactions with the white community in general. In Huntsville, the gifted and affable Harold Fanning Drake, having just finished an internship at Harlem Hospital, called on Dr. Kates, the newly arrived white doctor in nearby Madison. The two sat talking on a front yard swing at the widow's house where Kates had taken temporary quarters. Suddenly, the widow motioned to Kates to come to the door and told him, "You'll have to take that Negro to the back porch." When Kates protested, arguing that Drake was a doctor just like him, she said, "That has nothing to do with it."[24]

In a few cases, forging bonds of mutual support involved working with a white practitioner who was in trouble with his peers. During his Pascagoula practice, Barefield-Pendleton received a visit from a local white doctor who was being shunned by his colleagues: "He had a clinic, and he came by my office and asked me would I assist him in surgery. He said, 'Now, if you work with me, they are probably gonna get against you.'" Barefield-Pendleton never explained what the white doctor had done to warrant such ostracism by his white colleagues or by the local white community in general, only that the doctor in question had a pay telephone in his office because the telephone company would not give him a telephone. In the same vein, Anniston's Dr. Sherrer, unable to convince any of the white doctors in town to cover for him when he was out of town, found a solution: "There was a doctor that was recovering from alcoholism. Nobody wanted to cover for him, and we kind of scratched each other's back."[25]

Cultivating ties with just two or three white surgeons and obstetricians seems to have sufficed for most Black doctors. In Montgomery, Underwood developed bonds with three surgeons, which "was about all that I needed." In Mobile, Eyston A. Hunte tried "to carve out a relationship with those that I needed. I found a couple of surgeons who did work that I liked and that I liked to work with. I operated with many of them before I settled on those that I would refer to." Mobile's Walker B. LeFlore followed a similar course: "I would refer patients to doctors who were willing to communicate with me regarding my patients. That was essential. Doctors who were not willing to communicate would not get my patients."[26]

Not all Black physicians sought out such professional relationships. Though dependent on white specialists at St. Jude Hospital in Montgomery, the only place where she could admit patients, Hagalyn Seay Wilson managed to maintain a practice centered almost wholly within the Black community. That meant that she had no professional links to the local medical establishment: "I knew that there were certain people who had voted to keep me off the county medical society. I knew that there were eight white female physicians here. I only knew them by name. Many of them I never saw until a few years ago when one white female physician came to town and had a Christmas gathering and invited all the female physicians in town. That was the first time I had ever been to any integrated social affair with the white female physicians."[27]

PATTERNS OF AFRICAN AMERICAN MEDICAL PRACTICE

Anniston dentist Gordon A. Rodgers Jr., whose physician father had opened a medical office and drugstore in the town in 1924, recalled the informality that had governed the practice. The consultation room, he said, was just "a room in the drugstore, accessible to anybody coming in. There wasn't any real waiting room. I never heard of appointments at that time. I don't think he had any hours." In short, sick people just came to see his father when they could get off from work, "if they had a job."[28]

By the 1950s, certain elements of that system remained, as can be seen in Dr. Curry's description of his Birmingham practice: "It was walk-in. At that particular time, there were very few people who were insured. You did not have sick days or vacation days. The time that frequently most Black people could come to the doctor's office was after they had been to work that day, because they would need the transportation to get to and from work, and if they had a family member, they had to wait for the family member [to come home] so they could pick him up and bring him back to the doctor's office.

This meant that the doctor's office hours were very strange, all day and then way into the night—quite often eight, nine, or ten o'clock at night. We had Saturday [hours] and quite often Sunday by appointment."[29]

Though the office was essential for doing physical examinations and laboratory work, it was not where Black doctors spent the bulk of their time. "We would get up in the morning before office hours and make house calls," Curry said. "The people would ask you to stop by—can you see me at such-and-such a time in the morning? Sometimes, you were called out of your office. You'd take several hours, then come back to your office, leave your office at night and make another house call. This would happen quite often, especially during a flu epidemic."[30]

In Montgomery, Dr. Underwood was sometimes able to get in as many as ten early morning house calls before arriving at St. Jude Hospital at eight o'clock. The facility was part of a Catholic school and social services center for Black people, and it was the only place where Black physicians had hospital privileges. After making his rounds, Underwood would head off to his office: "I'd probably have house calls to make in the middle of the day, during my break, and at the end of the day." Nor did the demands cease once he came home: "As a matter of fact, during the years that I was making house calls, I really never felt comfortable putting on my pajamas until after midnight." His phone, he said, was always listed, and when he got called, he always went: "And a lot of people would call you to come to their homes because they didn't have cab fare. And most of the time, they wouldn't pay you either."[31]

In South Pittsburg, Dr. Moore usually got up at five o'clock and arrived at his office at six. "I'd make house calls and office visits, and then, between my office [hours]—say, twelve and three or twelve and four—I would make house calls. Sometimes, I'd leave the office and make house calls according to how bad it was. I was the youngest doctor here. Most of the [white] doctors were kind of elderly, and they didn't like to make night calls. I was the onliest doctor they could find. And back in them days, you had to make a lot of house calls over bad roads." Moore's record, he said, was 102 patients and two deliveries during a twenty-four-hour period, both deliveries being at home.[32]

Several other doctors in the oral accounts recall days when they saw up to a hundred patients. It was a remarkable feat when one considers that in 2020 primary care physicians were typically treating between twenty and twenty-five patients a day while maintaining a patient file or "panel" of around 2,500. To be sure, some Black physicians tried to maximize the number of people they saw as a way to offset their low fees. As Barefield-Pendleton put it, "If I just had a volume of patients and did the work, money would come as a result."[33]

In Anniston, Dr. Sherrer went further, allocating no more than ten minutes per patient, a goal sometimes frustrated by those having the temerity to ask questions about their care. Black teachers, in his view, were the worst: "They'll come and ask me questions that they should have asked their specialist. They have lists, like on a pad, twenty things, and it'll take you four or five times longer to see that patient."[34]

The large numbers of patients that Black doctors typically examined over a twenty-four-hour period often included whole families. Because many Black women found it hard to get time off from their employers, they sometimes brought along family members to the doctor's office, from aging parents to children with stomach or ear aches. House calls were no different. During the flu epidemic of 1957, Dr. Hereford got a call to the home of sharecroppers living on a farm owned by Senator John Sparkman, where both husband and wife had the flu and where their nine children were suffering from bronchitis or sore throats and were just developing the flu: "I examined every single person in that family on a house call and gave them all injections and what I used to call a family bottle of medicine." Meanwhile, residents of Black neighborhoods often recognized Hereford's car, and one or two might be waiting outside to ask him to stop by and see an ailing mother or grandparent.[35]

After several years of practice, Hereford settled into a routine in which he was seeing forty-five to fifty patients a day, plus a dozen or so others once he was permitted to practice in the Black ward of Huntsville Hospital. At some point, he counted up the charts in his office, and there were around eleven thousand names: "Of course, some of those patients had moved out of town, some had become inactive, and some of them had expired. Still, I think my active load of patients was somewhere in the neighborhood of six thousand. Most of the family practitioners I knew had two thousand or three thousand patients."[36]

Though fewer Black physicians in the country as a whole identified as general practitioners, 88 percent of the doctors in our group regarded themselves as such. A 1967 survey found that while 73 percent of those belonging to the NMA were involved in patient care, just 39 percent described themselves as primary care physicians; others limited their practices to internal medicine, obstetrics, pediatrics, and other fields.

Nationally, 22 percent of NMA members had achieved board certification in a specialty by 1967. By contrast, just 2.5 percent of Alabama's Black physicians had been able to do so, and even these were forced to treat a broad spectrum of complaints in order to make a living. This state of affairs, said Tuskegee surgeon Thomas J. Calhoun, "was more or less forced upon you. If you are working in a small town and you're a doctor, the patients don't care what your specialty is. They want to see a doctor."[37]

In Montgomery County, home to sixty-four thousand Black residents, doctors Winston and Pryor had little choice but to incorporate primary care into their surgical practice. That included home visits. "We would spend Saturday evenings, sometimes Sundays, making house calls," Winston said. "Very low money in that, almost none, but it was a service that you rendered." While they treated "a lot of the economically secure teachers and other [middle-class] Blacks," he and Pryor also cared for some of the poorest in the city: "We saw all comers, with or without money, and most of them didn't have money." Oklahoma native Calvin R. Johns Jr., who joined the practice in 1969, remembered that the sick came from as far as fifty miles away: "We had patients from up in Millbrook, up in Tallassee, Tuskegee, Union Springs. We had people from Lowndes County, Autauga, and Butler counties, from down in Greenville."[38]

In making house calls, Dr. Winston prepared himself for all contingencies: "You carried your bag, hoping that you could treat [the sick] at home. We had medicine for pain. We had antibiotics. We had medicines for asthma and things that we could sew up a cut with. We had just a variety of what you thought would be the common thing you could take care of at home—debride ulcers, do minor surgery, open abscesses. I mentioned asthmatic attacks because we saw a lot of those at home."[39]

The realization that a doctor could not confine his practice to a specialty dawned on Dr. Underwood soon after he began. His plan had been to focus exclusively on internal medicine and cardiology, but that did not last long. His son, also an internist, later recalled the story his father had told him. One day, a woman who was nine months pregnant showed up to ask if he would deliver her baby. At first he declined, telling her that she needed to see an obstetrician. She replied that the white obstetrician she visited had told her, "Y'all have a colored doctor in town. You go to him." Underwood agreed to deliver the baby, the first of many in his practice.[40]

In time, Underwood grew accustomed to his role as both a specialist and a family practitioner, to the point that when patients called his home wanting him to come out, he no longer asked what was wrong: "I was called one night, and when I got there, this lady was having a baby at her house. The baby was on the way out. Had no choice but to deliver it there at home. And, of course, I never heard from her again."[41]

Most Black physicians followed unwritten guidelines as to which patients would be charged. Typically, doctors treated each other free of charge, and some, like Barefield-Pendleton, made a point of never charging Black nurses. Extended family members were sometimes treated for free, though this could be a problem when distant relatives showed up. At the top of the list were ministers. Dr. Sherrer remarked that of all the Black professionals, the minister "could have been the less educated, but he was the one that was gonna do the eulogy. He was looked up to. And it's the Black church that kept the Blacks together in slavery. So when they come [for treatment], don't dun them. If you do that, when they get up to do their sermon, [they might say], 'Oh, Dr. Sherrer sent me a bill.' And that's filtered through the whole community."[42]

As both a cardiologist and general practitioner, Dr. Montgomery charged five dollars for an office visit during the late 1950s, as opposed to the three dollars being asked by Birmingham's other Black doctors. Despite warnings from his colleagues that he would starve at those rates, he soon had a thriving practice, even though he had to carry a large nonpaying clientele, which he estimated to be around 40 percent of the practice. The fact that many of his patients had jobs in mining and steel-making helped to offset his losses; patients belonging to the United Mine Workers, for example, had health insurance, which meant that they could afford both office visits and prescriptions.[43]

In Roosevelt City, southwest of the city, Barefield-Pendleton found that part of his clientele consisted of maids working "over the mountain" for five dollars a day. The term referred to the wealthiest sections of the city south of Red Mountain, including Homewood and Mountain Brook, whose inhabitants lived in isolation from the city's poor: "I was charging five dollars when I came here. I had some patients that I examined, they paid me, and I gave the money back to 'em because they didn't have any money to buy the drugs." Still, having a large patient base ensured him a modest gross income each year, which he remembered as being around $15,000 by the late 1950s.[44]

In Huntsville, Dr. Hereford characterized his practice as 20 percent nonpaying, 40 percent partially paying, and 40 percent fully paying: "If the patient had no cash, and if he didn't have Blue Cross—and only maybe 5 percent had Blue Cross—there was no way you were gonna be paid." Hereford knew the occupations of his patients and had a rough idea of what maids and janitors and detail men at the car dealerships were making, and he decided never to charge more for an office visit than a patient earned in a single day, though it was usually less. Even then, some patients had no money to fill their prescriptions, in which case he would give them free samples or, in desperate cases, tell them to charge their medicine to his drugstore account.[45]

On occasions, Hereford's colleague Harold Fanning Drake would likewise pay the pharmacy costs of indigent patients, to the dismay of his wife, Geneva Drake. When he began his practice in 1948, the fee for an office visit was three dollars, but, in her words, "If you gave him a pitiful story, you didn't have to pay. Oh, honey, yes—the people, their dogs, their fish, their grandchildren, feet, anything that hurt you, and he'd get up out of the bed and go see somebody." She told the story of a young woman with tuberculosis: "Harold got her into [treatment]. I think it was over in Decatur. [Later], she got to come home. She had a prescription. She didn't have [any money], and Harold was ordering her medicine. We kept it at the office. One day, the bill came in from the drugstore. I just had a fit. I said, 'She is not my child.' But he paid for it."[46]

In Montgomery, Underwood started off charging three dollars for an office visit. House calls were five dollars and, at night, seven dollars. "I might have seen seventy patients in one day," he said, "and ten of them might pay the whole bill. Over 50 percent probably wouldn't pay anything." At such times, Underwood would recall Dr. Adair's advice: "He told me, 'Jeff, if you find a patient who can't pay, you know he can't pay, just don't charge him, because the worst thing that could happen is that if you charge him and he can't pay, he won't ever say, 'I went to another doctor because I couldn't pay Dr. Underwood.' He'll say 'Dr. Underwood didn't treat me right. He couldn't diagnose my problem.' So I remembered that. And it just never mattered. I knew they couldn't pay. I was making a good living, I thought. I did it by seeing so many patients."[47]

Few Black doctors surpassed the compassion and generosity of Hagalyn Seay Wilson. Many who came seeking her help did so at the urging of her father, Rev. Solomon S. Seay Sr. She saw them all, maintaining a walk-in practice whose patients were exclusively Black: "They were poor—I would say that I had very few middle-income Black people. Maybe at least 30 percent were unable to pay." Wilson explained, "Making a lot of money was never a goal of mine, and so I probably didn't notice as long as I was able to pay my bills and keep my children in school and pay my taxes." The sheer volume of Wilson's patients ensured her a gross income of around $15,000 by 1960. Years later, her children recalled how many of their mother's patients would come to the house bearing gifts of fresh fruit and vegetables, and how, when the children grew up and left for college, they were all able to pack handmade quilts given to their mother as payment.[48]

At one point, Wilson was seeing up to one hundred patients a day in both office visits and house calls. Later, she began reserving two days a week to visit homebound patients. That meant hours of driving, usually within a forty-mile radius of Montgomery and sometimes all the way to Troy in adjoining Pike County, where she would stop by the Black hamlets, like the aptly named community of Needmore. She remembered that many of the homes had no soap and running water: "People dying for lack of attention—there was more of that at that time. We saw more far advanced malignancies, people who just didn't come to the doctor because they didn't have money, and when they did come it was too late for anybody to do anything about it."[49]

Like Wilson, our doctors witnessed firsthand the physical disorders affecting African American families. Heading the list was infant mortality. In Alabama's cities, for example, Black infant mortality was roughly twice that of white infants. Figure 3.3 depicts Black and white infant deaths in Jefferson County in 1944, including Birmingham proper and the industrial suburbs of Bessemer and Fairfield.

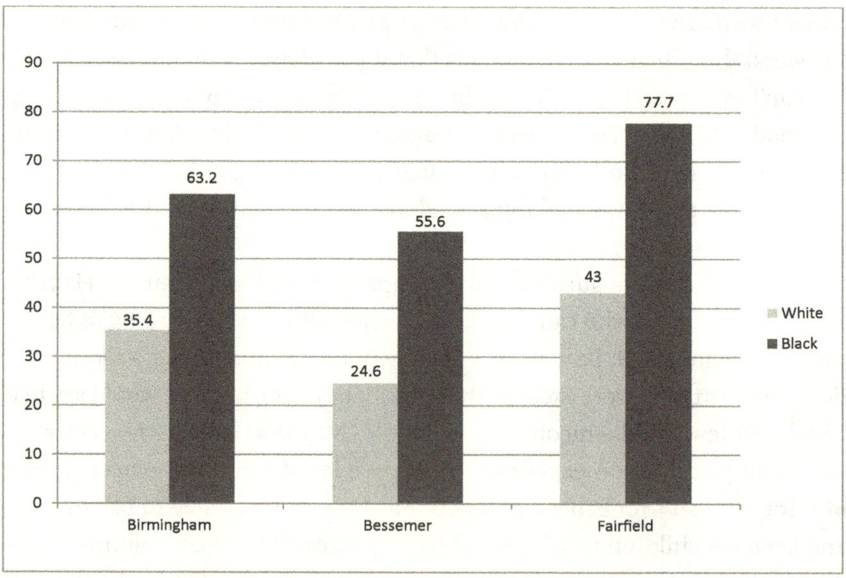

Figure 3.3. Black and white infant mortality per thousand births in Jefferson County, Alabama, 1944. (Jefferson County Board of Health, "The Public Health of Birmingham and Jefferson County" [1944], UAB Archives, 5.35 MC53.)

In Huntsville, Hereford recalled seeing "a lot of TB, a lot of syphilis, a lot of pneumonia, a lot of bronchitis." There were ear infections and gastroenteritis among children during the winter months and, among adults, metabolic diseases such as thyroid disorders and "a whole lot of diabetes."[50] Several oral histories allude to high rates of asthma, a disease that afflicted Black people with greater force than white people and whose causes included environmental conditions and airborne allergens.

In South Pittsburg, Dr. Moore treated "a lot of tuberculosis and emphysema. There's a cement plant down here, and they had these foundries where they breathe this dust. And then, these coal mines up there. They called it chronic obstructed [pulmonary] disease—COPD. That's on account of people working in the dust and all. They just couldn't breathe." Over time, Moore gained a reputation as the town's "emphysema doctor," which meant only that he had more emphysema patients than anybody else "because these are older people that you can't cure, and nobody else wanted to be bothered with them. About all you could do was give them a bronchial dilator, something to make 'em breath better."[51]

Hypertension was rampant among African Americans in the state, and whether its victims lived or died often depended on how much money they had. "Everybody had high blood pressure," Dr. Montgomery recalled. "By everybody, I mean 40 to 60 percent of a certain age. They took all the home remedies. They'd taken garlic for their high blood pressure. They'd taken everything from axle grease to whatever you want to name."

Montgomery remembered how poor people without health insurance would get their prescriptions but could not afford to buy enough medicine to last a full month: "So you prescribe sixty pills, one twice a day. They got half of them and made 'em last a month." Things improved only with Medicare and Medicaid. "When I first started practicing medicine, I pronounced people [dead] who had strokes, hemorrhages of the brain, all the time. After 1970, when Medicaid came into this state, the number of people who died of massive strokes decreased markedly. I saw it in my own practice, because they could get the medicine."[52]

Both Black and white patients benefitted from an array of lifesaving treatments available by the 1950s, from sulfa drugs and penicillin to vaccines for tetanus, pertussis, and polio. But not everyone shared equally in these breakthroughs. Dr. Moore, for example, noted that a serum was available for pneumonia but that a country doctor could not use it: "You had four types of pneumonia, and you had to get the type of pneumonia before you could get a serum. I don't mean vaccine: it was a serum. Well, you see, that was off-limits to me 'cause there wasn't no way in the world for me to get the lab results to get the types of pneumonia they had."

The same obstacles characterized Moore's treatment of children's disease: "I've seen a whole lot of whooping cough and chicken pox and measles, seen 'em all. But see, I lost some kids with the whooping cough because their parents weren't able to pay for the vaccine. So they just didn't give 'em a shot. Back in those days, you had to pay for shots to keep from having whooping cough and diphtheria."[53]

Added to the demands on a doctor was the all-consuming task of delivering babies, which, when one includes time spent on prenatal care, might occupy up to 40 percent of one's practice. When Wilson began practicing in Montgomery, she estimated that the three active Black physicians in the city were together doing one hundred deliveries a month: "Their offices were very, very crowded with patients in the halls as well as in the waiting rooms."[54] Toward the end of their careers, some of our doctors were able to cite the number of deliveries they had performed—2,000 by Wilson in Mobile, 2,200 by Hereford in Huntsville, "half by lamplight and one on a Trailways bus." Hereford estimated that for every 500 Black babies born in Madison County during the 1950s, he and Dr. Drake delivered 200; white doctors delivered 150; and midwives did the rest. According to Hereford, there were two dozen trained and licensed Black midwives in the county—the only ones with whom he would deal—plus three or four dozen "self-proclaimed midwives," usually relatives or elderly women.[55]

Black doctors generally maintained good relations with midwives and were available to help if problems developed with the delivery—a breech birth, for example, or an umbilical cord wrapped around the infant's leg or arm. Stanley Hand, a white physician who began practicing in Athens, west of Huntsville, in 1950, recalled that the most frequent problem for which he was called to help out midwives was excessive bleeding caused by a retained placenta.

In 1940, 73 percent of white births and more than 90 percent of Black births in Alabama were at home. Twenty years later, the figures had dropped to 3 percent and 46 percent, respectively. As more Black mothers chose to be delivered in hospitals, the number of midwives who had been approved by county boards of health declined from 3,000 in 1930 to 2,600 in 1940 to fewer than 100 in 1980.[56] Still, midwifery died hard in rural areas. Growing up in the Black Belt, future obstetrician Charles E. McGruder remembered that though there was a Black physician in Greensboro, "as poor as everybody was—everybody I knew was poor—you wouldn't be going to try and get a doctor to come out there and pay him all that money from thirteen or fourteen miles when a midwife would be able to deliver a baby."[57]

Physicians who were called to a home delivery might spend hours of waiting during the mother's labor. Spouses of doctors with nursing degrees sometimes helped out, as in the case of Geneva Drake. "We sort of worked as a team with deliveries," she recalled. "One January, we had twenty-one deliveries. Of course, I knew about OBGYN, being a public health nurse. Sometimes, we would have three in labor, and he would go on one, and I'd go on one, and whoever got through would go to the other."[58]

On one occasion, Geneva Drake accompanied her husband to the home of white sharecroppers in rural Tennessee, north of Huntsville, to deliver a baby. They were met at around 8:30 a.m. by several white men in a truck who drove them through a succession of gates until they reached the house. Inside, the expectant mother was just starting to go into labor, which meant that Geneva Drake and her husband had to occupy themselves while the men went back to the fields. By dinnertime, the baby still had not arrived, and the couple shared a meal of cornbread, greens, and potatoes with their hosts, everyone holding hands as a blessing was offered. Geneva Drake recalled that it was about 9:00 or 10:00 p.m. before they got home after finally delivering the baby.[59]

Except for the occasional white person in the waiting room hoping to persuade a Black doctor to prescribe pain pills—or, as sometimes happened, a white deacon or Sunday school teacher looking for antibiotics following an out-of-town tryst—African Americans made up the bulk of a Black doctor's practice. There were a few exceptions. Hereford estimated Dr. Drake's patients to be about 10 percent white. In Fayetteville, Latha M. Donalson enjoyed popularity among both races, his widow recalling that "he had a mixed practice all through the years."[60] In Anniston, Dr. Sherrer catered to even larger numbers of white patients, who eventually constituted 90 percent of his practice. His modest fees, combined with a brief experiment using acupuncture to treat obesity (which got him into trouble with local and state medical authorities), attracted numerous Appalachian white people, many coming from the six predominantly white counties that formed part of Sand Mountain in northeast Alabama.

Dr. Moore's tenure in South Pittsburg was the longest and most successful example of a mixed-race practice. While he had resolved early on never to let himself be insulted by racist remarks from a patient, he had to be cautious. One night, he got a call for help from the husband of a white woman in labor:

> This was out in Sweetens Cove. The water was up, and you had to go a long ways around and come back in another way and walk a certain distance. Apparently, I was the only doctor he could find who would do it 'cause that's the first time I had seen the woman. But I knew her daddy, and I had doctored her daddy. When I got there, her daddy was there and her husband, and she saw me, and she said, 'Is that all you could find?' He said, 'Yeah.' She said, 'Well, I don't want him.'
>
> So I started [to leave]. I went through the kitchen 'cause that's the way they were going in. That's one time I went through the back because the front porch had so much junk on it. I said, 'I'll tell you something. She's gonna need a doctor.'
>
> Her daddy and her husband said, 'No, you ain't gonna leave. You just stay around here. Don't you go nowhere.' I'd started out, and they said, 'No, come back. Come back.' We sat down out there and talked. And she was having pains in there, and after a while, she said, 'Where is he?' That lady got pregnant three more times, and she came to me for prenatal care. And I delivered three more children for her, and the children are still around here.[61]

ANNUAL EARNINGS

Before Medicare and Medicaid, Black physicians often had trouble making ends meet. Census reports and NMA surveys provide a rough idea of where the incomes of African American practitioners in Alabama stood in relation to those of white doctors. In 1959, at a time when American families were earning around $5,600 a year ($50,000 in 2020 dollars), the median income for physicians as a group was $15,000 ($134,000). That for nonwhite physicians (three-fourths in this category were African Americans) stood at $6,000 ($54,000). In short, nonwhite doctors earned less than half of what their white counterparts earned.[62]

Black physicians in the South tended to trail their counterparts in other areas of the country, though the introduction of Medicare in 1965 helped to improve the situation. A survey of NMA members taken four years later showed that just over 46 percent of those in the South were now earning between $20,000 and $40,000. An additional 27 percent made over $40,000. That left about 27 percent earning below $20,000. Taxes, overhead, and operating costs, plus the hiring of office staff, took a large share of the doctor's earnings.[63]

In Huntsville, Hereford kept a record of his income during his first two years of practice; in 1957, he took in gross receipts of around $20,000, out of which came medical and office supplies, rent, telephone, janitorial services, and gas and oil for the car. The latter was considerable, given the thousands of miles he put on his Oldsmobile making house calls. The result was a profit of around $7,800 ($72,000), a figure that would have been lower had not his wife, Martha Ann Hereford, who had trained as a nurse, worked in the office that year doing paperwork, giving injections, taking blood and urine samples, and assisting in home deliveries.[64]

Though not driven by the religious convictions motivating Hagalyn Seay Wilson, Dr. Moore was likewise indifferent to wealth. He sometimes received fresh food from patients but insisted that these were gifts rather than payments: "I never did send no statements. I just doctored everybody that come in there, whether they had the money or not. I just left it to them to pay. They'd give me chickens and things like that, but nobody never did pay me like that. I had a fellow to pay me with squirrels and rabbits, but that was by request."[65]

Other Black physicians were more calculating. "One of the weirdest practices" in Birmingham during the 1950s, Barefield-Pendleton reported, was that of Lorenzo S. Demby, who configured his schedule to fit shift changes in local industries. Demby "practiced all night, slept all day. He had a driver and would come in at about six o'clock in the morning and go to bed, and then he'd stay in his office until eleven o'clock at night, and his office was full." Barefield-Pendleton believed that the most successful Black doctor in the city was a member of a prominent family named Adolphus W. Plump, who treated industrial workers in Bessemer and well-to-do Black residents in the North Titusville area where his office was located: "I guess people owed him more money than any doctor. One month, he had a delivery every day, plus all his practice."[66]

Dr. Montgomery was among the highest earners of the state's Black specialists. He recalled that when he started practicing in 1958, his wife's teaching salary was about $400 a month: "She had surmised if I could make $400 a month, that would give us $800 a month. And the first month I practiced I made, I think, a gross of $1,300. Dr. Hampton Brewer had told me, 'You'll make about $1,300 or $1,400 your first month,' and that's exactly what I made. [After three years], I think it had got into the twenties or thirties [annually]. We really did not make any money in the practice of medicine—I mean, good income—until Medicare came into being."[67]

Here and there one finds individuals who followed the path of the state's early Black physician-entrepreneurs. An example was Oliver S. Gumbs of Mobile, one of ten physicians of Caribbean origins in our group. He completed his training at Meharry in 1941 and after practicing in Huntsville moved to Mobile in order to join the staff of Martin de Porres Hospital, a Catholic facility that opened in April 1950.

Besides overseeing an expanding practice, Gumbs launched a profitable business career in real estate and banking, helping to create the first savings bank for Black residents in the city.[68] In addition, he was a founding member of the Mobile branch of Kappa Alpha Psi, a predominantly Black fraternity specializing in education and social issues. In later years, the group elected him Grand Polemarch, or chief executive officer, a position he used to provide scholarships and after-school programs for Black children. In May 1981, *Ebony* magazine included Gumbs on its annual list of "the 100 most influential Black Americans."

By this point, Gumbs was operating two medical offices in the city, one on St. Anthony Street, west of center city, and the other in the heavily Black northern suburb of Prichard. With implementation of Medicaid in Alabama in 1970, the latter began attracting large numbers of patients from the area's impoverished neighborhoods. Soon, the stress of juggling his business and medical practices began to overwhelm the aging doctor, and in 1973 he invited a recent Howard graduate named Eyston A. Hunte, a native of Anguilla who was just finishing an internship at Freedmen's, to come to Mobile and work with him. "He said he was getting older," Hunte recalled. "He had this big practice in Mobile, [and] he would like somebody to join him because he was slowing down."

Hunte soon discovered that his employer had a passion for secrecy: "Dr. Gumbs was a businessman, and I don't know if he was always that way, but in the latter part of his life he was consolidating his money and trying to get as much of it as he could. He hated banks. He kept his money in cash in a box under his bed. He paid me once a month by pulling out a roll of twenty-dollar bills or hundred-dollar bills and peeling them off." After a year, Hunte decided that he did not wish to work for Gumbs any longer but agreed to remain in the Prichard office.

During the 1980s, the IRS accused Gumbs of failing to file income taxes for the years 1977–1980, thereby avoiding payments totaling $70,000. According to press reports, the assistant US attorney who prosecuted the case also claimed that the doctor had evaded taxes in several of his real estate dealings and that he had misled IRS investigators in saying that all his medical receipts were in his patient and ledger cards, when the doctor knew that many checks were missing. The jury returned a guilty verdict: Gumbs was sentenced to five years' probation, fined $5,000, and made to perform two hundred hours of community service. He was also ordered to pay all income tax owed to the government, along with interest and penalties.[69]

As noted earlier, the distrust that certain African Americans harbored against Black physicians affected the earnings of some in our group, an attitude that Dr. Montgomery ascribed to history: "White doctors' opinions were better. See, we had been taught through our whole history, from slavery on, that white was better than Black, and most of us had accepted that." Barefield-Pendleton was only one of many to encounter this attitude: "I had a patient I almost came to blows with in my office. The patient said, 'I don't have no confidence in Black doctors.' I said, 'Why are you sittin' up in the damned office then? Why don't you get outta here?'"[70]

In certain instances, a patient's distrust was justified, particularly in regard to elderly Black doctors who had spent their professional lives without opportunities to update their skills. In Mobile, Ophelia Burnett Northcross remembered that James A. Franklin had a poor reputation among Black women; citing the tragic experiences of her aunt, Northcross claimed that Franklin did not know how to do the gynecological procedure known as dilation and curettage, or the removal of the tissue lining of the uterus in cases of bleeding or following a miscarriage. Once she heard her mother say, "I don't go to a Black physician."[71]

In fact, throughout most of his career Franklin had enjoyed a good reputation within the Black community, not just for his medical services but for his efforts to get his sickest patients admitted to a white hospital. The problem was his insistence on continuing past his prime. When Walker B. LeFlore returned to Mobile in 1965, he found space on Davis Avenue in a building owned by the legendary physician, who had an office upstairs. Now approaching eighty, Franklin was struggling hard to keep up his old routines. The Black dentist Lawrence E. Carroll, an old family friend, recalled his last days: "Dr. Franklin had his medical route. I think he was the last of the home visitors. Even up until he was dying, he was making visits, especially out in the Plateau area, 'cause that's where he started."[72]

Franklin's second wife, Marguerite Franklin, witnessed the decline: "When he began to get feeble, I would take him on his calls. I would drive for him. I waited outside for him, but I would take his bag, because he was getting feeble, and put it on the porch, and somebody in the house would come and get it for him."[73]

Birmingham's Pierce S. Moten, who, as we shall see in the next chapter, spent his life fighting to improve health care for Black people, was another who refused to call it quits. As he entered his seventies, his colleagues began to recognize his limitations. "He should have been retired at the time that I met him," Barefield-Pendleton said, "which meant he was slipping, and he actually tried to carry on. And a lot of the young doctors, particularly Dr. [Robert] Stewart, would take his deliveries. [He] would go out and get these deliveries, and then, you know, he wouldn't be able to follow through. His speed just wasn't [there]."[74]

Barefield-Pendleton observed that anti-Black medical bias among African Americans was most evident in cases of surgery, especially those involving the eye. It was something that ophthalmologist Alexander Lee Brewer well understood. After finishing Meharry in 1944, Brewer completed an internship at Homer G. Phillips, followed by a residency in ophthalmology at Chicago's Cook County Hospital. He then returned to Birmingham and worked in general practice for two years before heading back north to pursue a residency in ophthalmology, in the process completing the prestigious Lancaster Course in Ophthalmology in Lewiston, Maine. Despite failing the pathology section in his first attempt to pass his boards, he overcame his deficiencies and in 1957 became a diplomate of the American Board of Ophthalmology and a fellow of the American Academy of Ophthalmology and Otolaryngology.

None of this mattered when Brewer set out to practice his specialty in Birmingham. Despite his best efforts, he ended up making only $2,000 or $3,000 a year. In his oral account, he related what happened: "It was sorta rough. In other words, if you really wanna know something, Blacks didn't have any confidence in a Black in a specialty. I was the first board-certified Black here, and, being in eye, they didn't have much confidence in me. So I suffered there."

Other Black doctors tried to help Brewer by referring patients to him, but most of the latter failed to show up after learning that he was Black or, having come into the office a few times, quietly left him for a white doctor. Brewer remembered one case in particular:

> I treated [a Black patient] about a year for glaucoma, and after about a year, I couldn't control the glaucoma on medication, and I told him, "Ah, looks like I can't control the glaucoma now, and so I think we better do some surgery."
>
> So the patient told me, "Oh, doctor, I don't want no surgery."
>
> I say, "Well, I can't throw you out in the street. So use this medication and come back and see me in two weeks." In two weeks, the patient didn't show up. A month, the patient didn't show up. Two months, the patient didn't show up.

> So one day I happened to see the patient down [at] the Masonic Temple going through the lobby. Only thing I said to him was good morning, but I never said anything to him about his eyes. After about a year, I heard that he was in the hospital being operated on for glaucoma. In other words, he had dumped me and gone to another physician.[75]

More Black board-certified physicians would have helped to allay this kind of prejudice, but this was not possible so long as they were barred from the hospitals. "I heard this from the mouths of many Black physicians," Curry said, "that if they would open the doors to that hospital today, I would be on the train tomorrow to do a residency."[76]

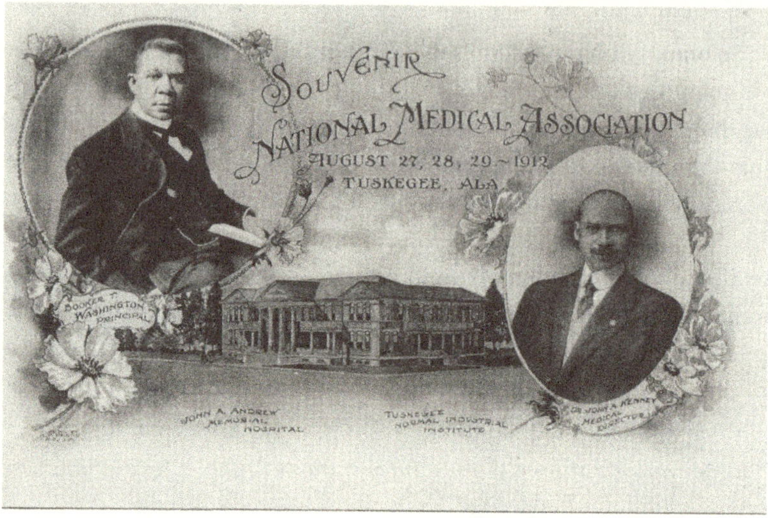

Figure Postcard commemorating 1912 meeting of the National Medical Association in Tuskegee. Symbolizing Tuskegee Institute's embrace of Black health care and the training of Black physicians as central to its mission, the postcard shows Booker T. Washington (1856–1915) on the left and Dr. John A. Kenney (1874–1950), director of the campus hospital, on the right. The new John A. Andrew Memorial Hospital, seen in the background, would be dedicated the following year. (Courtesy of the late Linda Kenney Miller, granddaughter of Dr. John A. Kenney.)

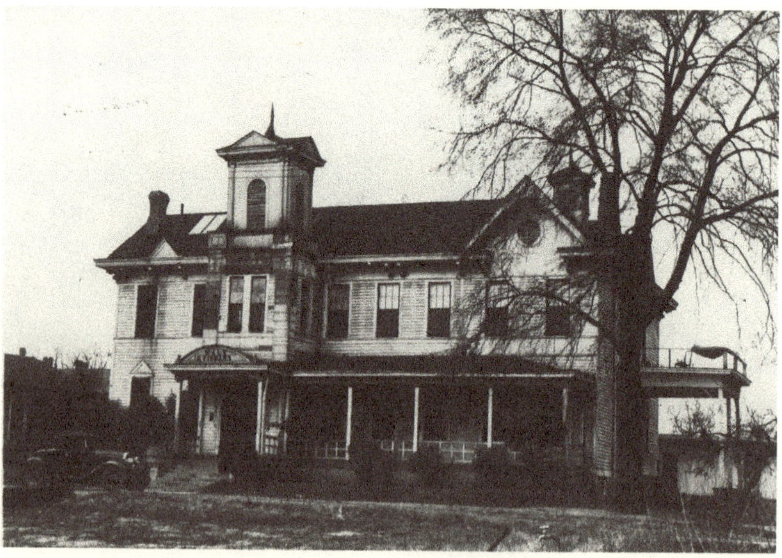

Hale Infirmary, Montgomery. Opened in 1890 through the efforts of Booker T. Washington's protégé, Dr. Cornelius Dorsette (1852?–1897), Hale Infirmary was the first hospital for African Americans in Alabama. (Alabama Department of Archives and History.)

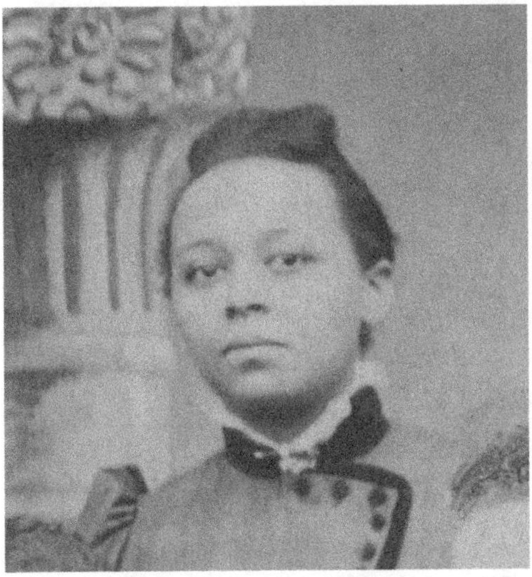

Dr. Halle Tanner Dillon. An 1891 honors graduate of the Woman's Medical College of Pennsylvania, Halle Tanner Dillon (1864–1901) accepted Booker T. Washington's offer of the post of school physician at Tuskegee Institute on condition that she pass the state's stringent licensing requirements. After a grueling ten-day examination, she passed with a score of 78.81, becoming the first woman of any race certified to practice medicine in Alabama. (Photo courtesy of Legacy Center, Drexel University, College of Medicine.)

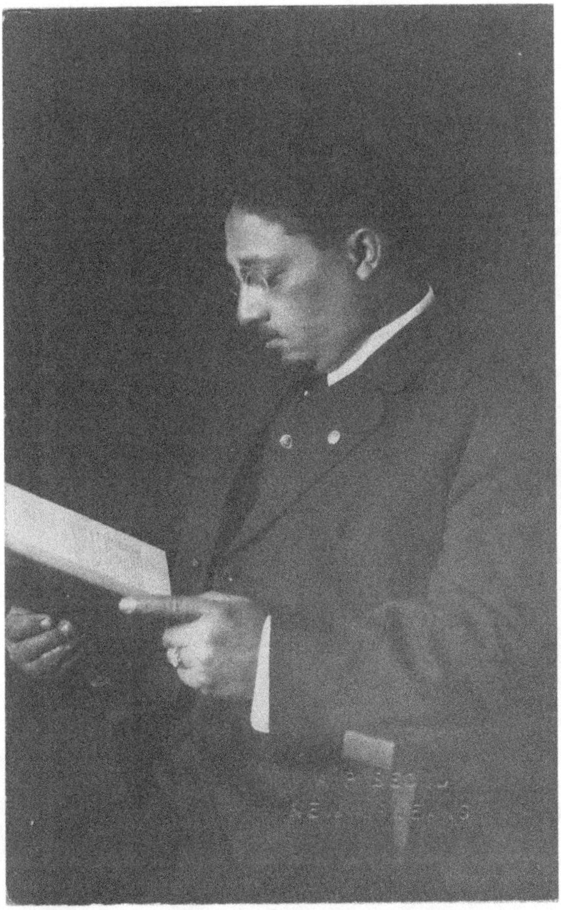

Dr. Arthur McKinnon Brown, ca.1932. Birmingham's distinguished Black surgeon Arthur McKinnon Brown (1867–1939) served as a contract physician in Cuba during the war with Spain in 1898 and later worked with Booker T. Washington in promoting health care for African Americans. According to one account, he chose to practice in Alabama because of the fearsome reputation of its medical licensure examinations. He scored an average of 87.8, reputed to have been among the highest ever earned to that point. (Alabama Department of Archives and History.)

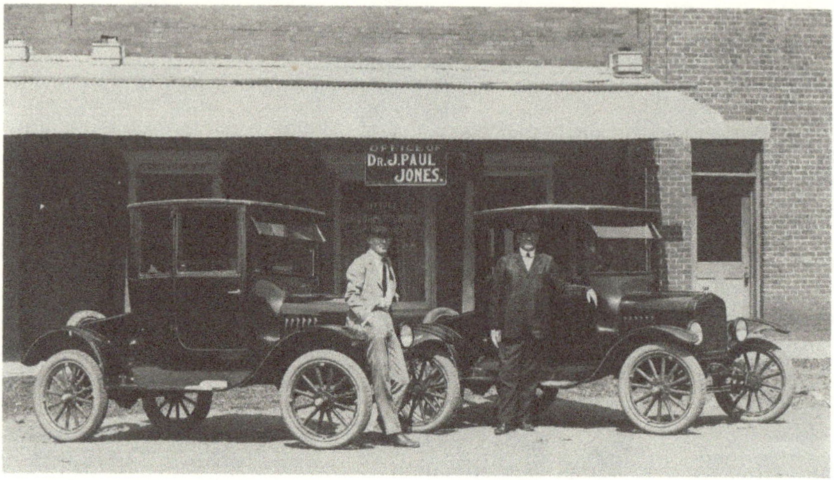

Separate waiting rooms for Black and white patients in rural Wilcox County, Alabama, ca.1920. Doctors J. Paul Jones, left, and Warburton Jones, right, stand next to their Model T automobiles at the entrance to their office in tiny Camden in the Black Belt. Doors on left and right designate entrances to separate waiting rooms for Black and white patients. According to an internal diagram, there were also separate examination rooms and laboratories for Black and white patients, though x-ray services appear to have been shared. (UAB Archives, University of Alabama at Birmingham.)

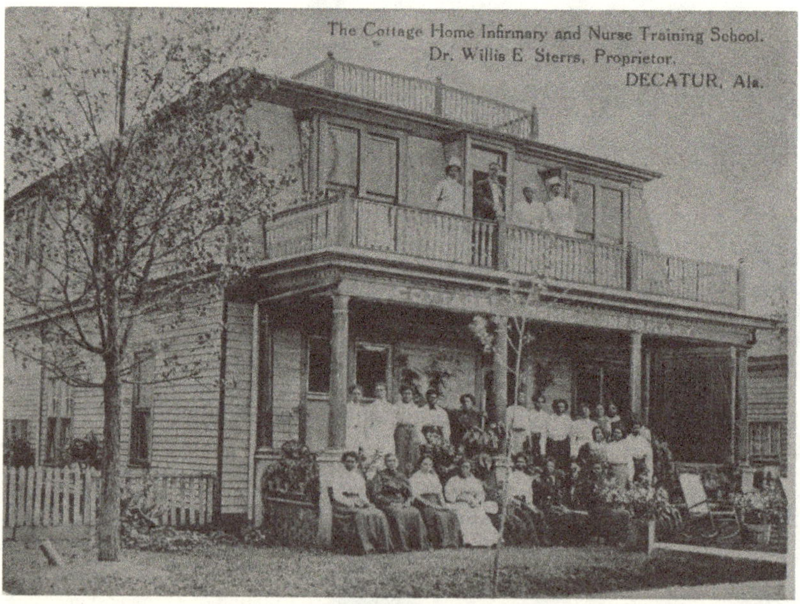

Cottage Home Infirmary and Nurse Training School, Decatur, 1913. Dr. Willis E. Sterrs (1867–1921) appears with his staff on the upper balcony of the Cottage Home Infirmary and Nurse Training School in Decatur in 1913 as nursing students pose on the porch below. (Memry Midgett Papers, African American Museum and Library at Oakland Public Library, Oakland, California.)

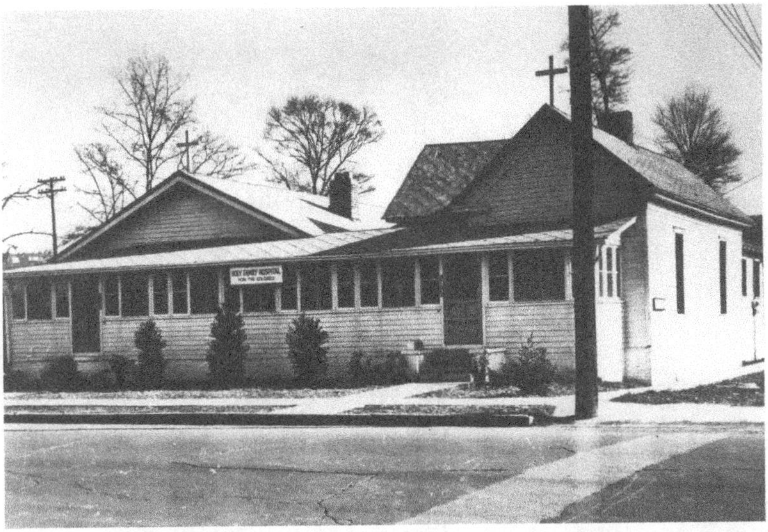

Holy Family Hospital, Birmingham, 1940s. Located in Ensley northwest of city center, Holy Family Hospital started off as a small maternity clinic operated by the Sisters of Charity of Nazareth, Kentucky. In 1943, the sisters expanded the facility by combining three dilapidated shotgun houses into one while using salvaged materials and plumbing fixtures. By 1948, the facility consisted of a twelve-bed ward and a staff of five sisters working alongside twenty-two Black doctors in the city. It was replaced in 1954 by a modern sixty-bed hospital. (UAB Archives, University of Alabama at Birmingham.)

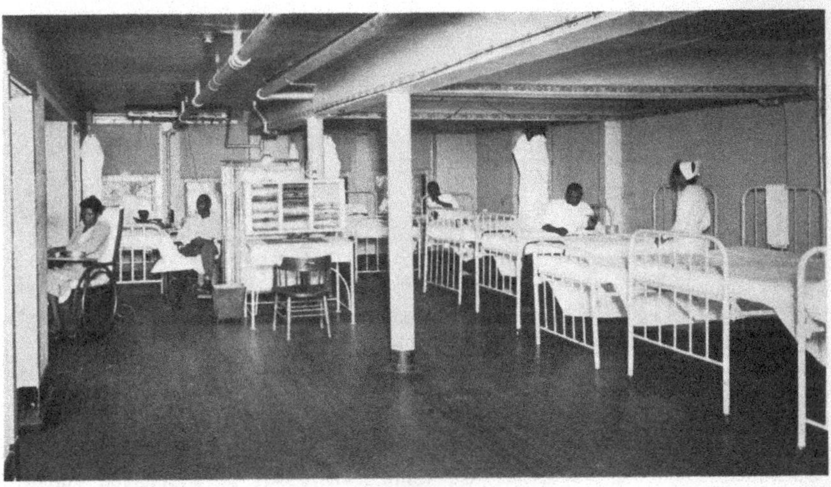

Black ward, South Highlands Infirmary, Birmingham, 1935. Board-certified ophthalmologist Alexander Lee Brewer long remembered the Black ward at South Highlands, where patients lay in the basement beneath the building's pipes: "You could visit your patients, but you couldn't treat them. You were just like any other visitor." (UAB Archives, University of Alabama at Birmingham.)

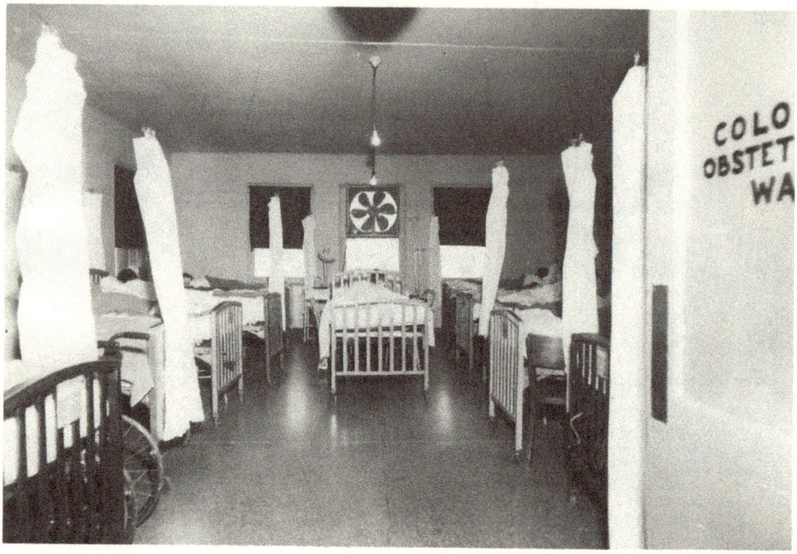

Black obstetrical ward, University Hospital, Birmingham, 1960s. Overcrowding and absence of privacy were not uncommon in the Black obstetrical wards of white hospitals. In Huntsville, Dr. Sonnie Wellington Hereford III remembered that the so-called colored wing "had one large room that served as our emergency room, delivery room, and operating room—what we called the ER, DR, and OR." (UAB Archives, University of Alabama at Birmingham.)

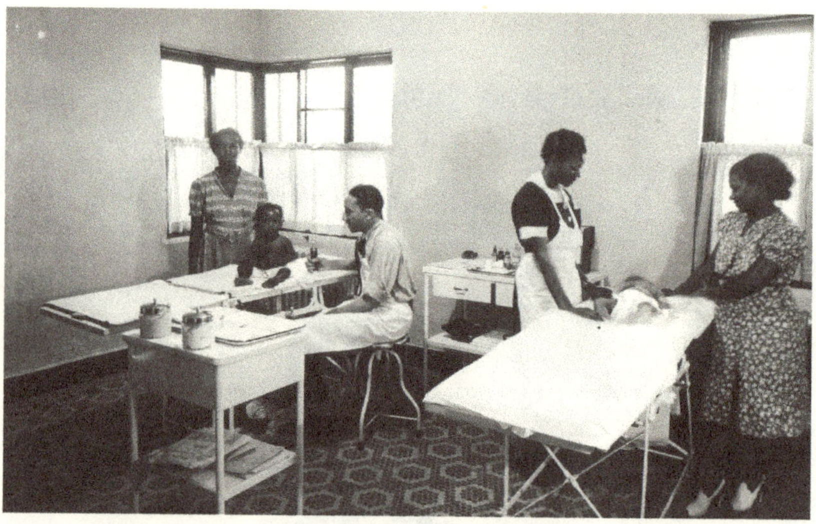

Black doctor examining baby at Slossfield Health Center, 1940s. The photograph is possibly that of Walter H. Maddux, a veteran of World War I who had done postgraduate training in pediatrics at the University of Chicago. In 1939, the Children's Bureau agreed to lend his services to the Slossfield Health Center, where he served as medical director while working to improve the lives of indigent Black families living in North Birmingham. (UAB Archives, University of Alabama at Birmingham.)

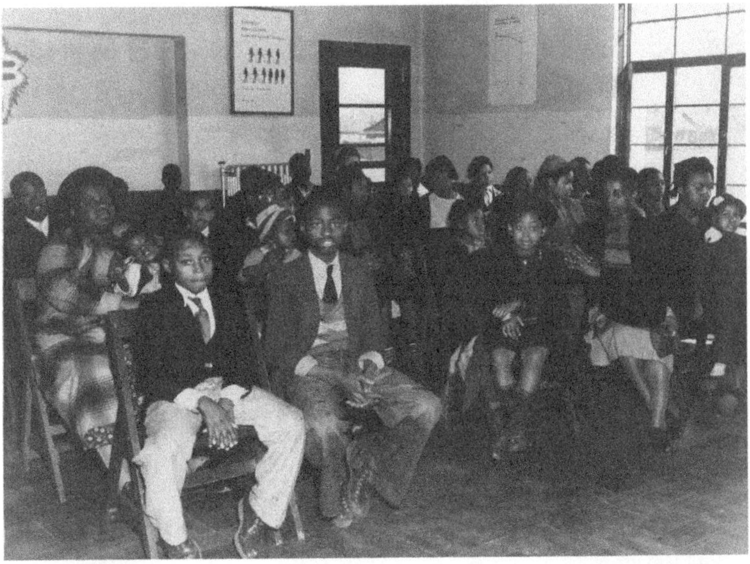

Children and parents attend a pediatric clinic at Slossfield Health Center, 1940s. The pediatric clinics at Slossfield focused on three areas: infant feeding, pediatric diagnosis, and immunizations. A sign on the wall next to the door notes that seven of ten Black children in Birmingham had received smallpox vaccinations, which may indicate that the clinic seen here dealt with immunizations. (UAB Archives, University of Alabama at Birmingham.)

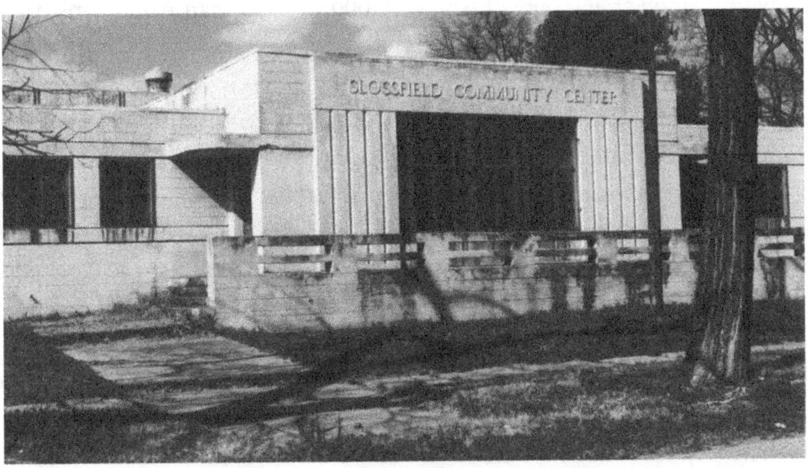

Slossfield Community Center, 2000. By 2000, the art deco buildings of the Slossfield Community Center, which sixty years earlier had won a national award as the most outstanding Black community center in the United States, lay in ruins, the trash and broken bottles scattered across the grounds serving as a complement to the discarded doors and desks stored inside. (Photo taken by author during a tour of Black medical sites in Birmingham on February 8, 2000, with Dr. Dodson M. Curry and UAB archivist Tim L. Pennycuff.)

CHAPTER FOUR

Birmingham's Black Doctors Fight for a Hospital of Their Own, 1930–1954

Despite its access to vast mineral deposits, Birmingham included some of the worst examples of health-care inequality in the state. As blast furnaces and sheet-metal mills began to dominate the landscape during the early years of the twentieth century, Birmingham's population had exploded, aided by Black convict labor from the coal mines, a form of industrial slavery. By 1930, the population stood at 260,000, of which 99,000 were African Americans, many of them working in unskilled, low-paying jobs in the new industries.[1]

The pioneering work of Dr. Pierce S. Moten, who in 1932 created a small but desperately needed maternal aid station that came to be known as the Southside Clinic, marked the start of a long campaign to provide a hospital for the city's African American doctors and their patients. Along with the care it provided to expectant mothers, the clinic helped pave the way for one of the most innovative medical endeavors in Alabama's history. Opened in 1939, the Slossfield Health Center received funding from the American Cast Iron Pipe Company (ACIPCO), the New Deal Works Progress Administration (WPA), the Julius Rosenwald Foundation of Chicago, and the Children's Bureau, which was created in 1912 for the protection of maternal and child welfare. The city's shutdown of the health center in 1948, followed by the failure of Black doctors to secure a place in the growing University of Alabama Medical Center downtown, laid bare the racist attitudes that governed the health care of African Americans and that delayed efforts to provide them access to modern, well-equipped hospitals.

One encouraging sign of progress was the expanding role of Catholic hospitals in providing African American doctors a place to practice. The building or enlargement of existing Catholic facilities introduced long-neglected moral and ethical values in dealing with the health-care crisis. Though limited to Birmingham, Mobile, Montgomery, and Selma, these hospitals represented the first small breach in the wall of segregation that had long prevented Black doctors from achieving professional equality.

HOSPITAL CARE FOR AFRICAN AMERICANS

The years following World War I saw a scattering of new clinics and nurse-training programs for Alabama's Black population, many of them created by fraternal orders such as the Knights of Pythias and its women's auxiliary, the Grand Court of the Order of Calanthe. As figure 4.1 shows, by 1937 Alabama ranked fifth in its number of Black hospitals among a sampling of eight Deep South states.

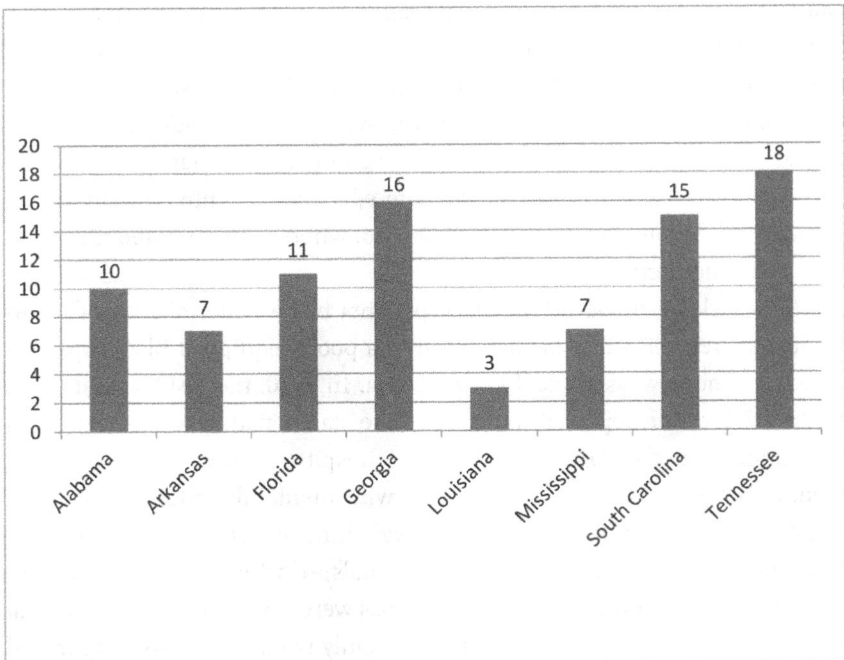

Figure 4.1. Black hospitals and nurse training schools operated by African Americans in Alabama and the Deep South, 1937 (national total = 180). (Numbers derived from Monroe N. Work [ed.], *Negro Year Book: An Annual Encyclopedia of the Negro 1937–1938*, Tuskegee Institute, AL: Negro Year Book Publishing Co., 290–92.)

The need for hospitals catering solely to Black people reflected the desperate choices confronting African Americans during the Jim Crow era. As a rule, the sick endured their suffering at home, nursed by a family member or friend and, if one could be afforded, visited occasionally by either a Black or a white physician. While home care was the rule, some emergencies demanded hospitalization, from appendicitis to fractures. "In the South," wrote Algernon Brashear Jackson in 1928, "colored pay patients go to the hospital chiefly for surgical, and seldom for medical care." Jackson, professor of public health at Howard, made the observation as part of a report commissioned by the AMA's Council on Medical Education and Hospitals. In all, he visited 120 Black hospitals, most of them in the South, including twelve in Alabama. Of the 120, he assigned a grade of "A" to just sixteen and recommended that twenty-seven be shut down.

Except for Hale Infirmary in Montgomery and Andrew Memorial in Tuskegee, the state's twelve Black hospitals were a sad testament to the care available to African Americans. While Jackson paid tribute to the doctors who had founded the first infirmaries, he was scathing in his criticisms of what some of these had become, accusing their directors of "untrained and ignorant management." He reserved special contempt for those who, in his judgment, were exploiting the labor of young Black women under the guise of offering a nursing education: "They cajole and persuade many little country and small town girls of most inadequate education to enter their 'training schools' and become 'nurses,' the majority of whom never rise above the dignity of glorified scrub women."[2]

While Jackson thought that Black patients had a better chance of recovery in a segregated white hospital than in a poorly equipped Black one, that choice was not always available in Alabama. In 1920, the AMA's Council on Medical Education reported that fifty of the state's sixty-seven counties had no hospital. A decade later, there were 115 hospitals, counting those for children, tuberculosis victims, and patients with mental disorders. In addition to a witches' brew of badly regulated private infirmaries, sanitoria, and poor asylums, there were seventy general hospitals, of which fifty-one were private and nineteen, public. Among both types were some that lacked x-ray machines, laboratories, and steam laundries. Only twenty-three were approved by the American College of Surgeons, of which just three, including Andrew Memorial in Tuskegee, were qualified to train interns.[3]

The percentage of white hospitals containing beds for Black patients throughout the state is unknown, consistent with patterns in other southern states whose hospital managers failed to document Jim Crow practices in their wards.[4] In absolute terms, according to one Black newspaper in Birmingham, there were only sixty-five hospitals in the whole of Alabama in 1941 that contained beds for Black patients.[5] As to the proportion of beds available to them, it is clear that in relation to their numbers, it was far inferior to that of white patients. Alfred W. Dent, president of Dillard University in New Orleans who had earlier served as superintendent of the city's Flint-Goodridge Hospital, placed the number of beds in Alabama at just 1,213 during the 1940s, at a time when African Americans numbered almost 947,000. White inhabitants, numbering 1,780,000, had access to 3,591 beds.[6]

Newspaper reports offer a glimpse of what these segregated wards were like. In the town of Enterprise, one hospital maintained an annex for Black patients in a field behind the main structure, to which it was connected by a dirt path; the annex was a wooden shack of four rooms that, in the words of a Black employee, had been "pulled up" to the main hospital in 1940, its walls bricked, and a partition added to provide more rooms and a bath. A Greenville hospital that opened in 1924 featured an annex for Black patients in the rear of the main building; its walls had diagonal boards covered with tar paper inside and weatherboarding outside and was warmed by one heater for twenty patients.[7]

Only slightly better off were Black wards that had been paid for by sources outside the state. When fundraising for a new hospital in Huntsville began during the early 1920s, Virginia McCormick, daughter of the inventor Cyrus McCormick, donated $50,000 to build a wing for Black patients, specifying that it be included as part of the main structure. While praising her generosity, Dr. Carl A. Grote, who in 1917 gained fame by stopping an outbreak of typhoid fever in the city, made it clear that Black patients and visitors in the new annex would be isolated from the main unit: "There will be separate entrances, separate halls, separate operating rooms, separate everything."[8]

Separate meant unequal. When the white pediatrician Richard L. Lester Jr. started practicing in Huntsville Hospital in the mid-1950s, he recalled "numerous times seeing cockroaches and mice and rats coming across the hallways" in the Black wing, which also lacked facilities for premature Black babies. On one occasion, an infant weighing just two and a half pounds was placed in an incubator and wheeled into a room with "an old fellow who had emphysema and chronic lung disease."[9]

By 1938, Birmingham, the state's largest city, had fourteen hospitals and 1,689 beds—about 3.5 per 1,000 inhabitants. A report published by the Jefferson County Medical Society indicated that almost 38 percent of the 41,000 patients treated that year were charity cases and that Hillman, the county hospital, had alone treated 19,000 patients, of which 86 percent were charity cases. The report further noted that all private pay hospitals were forced to turn away patients either because some could not afford treatment or because beds were unavailable.[10]

Lack of money and beds effectively summarized the dilemma faced by African Americans who had the misfortune of getting sick. In 1941, *The Weekly Review*, owned by the Black editor Robert Durr, estimated that the number of beds available to Birmingham's Black population was a mere 427, which included 17 provided by Children's Home, the only Black hospital at that time in the city: "One Negro hospital, 25 practicing Negro physicians and 102,292 Negro people whose health must be cared for. Somehow that just does not balance."[11]

Being denied admission to hospitals was just one part of the Black experience in a place touted by white residents as The Magic City. A white banker named Charles F. Zukoski Jr., who studied law at Harvard and later worked as a trust officer for the First National Bank in Birmingham, was an early supporter of a Black hospital and was stunned by the depths of racial animosity he found after moving to Birmingham from St. Louis in 1926. Inequality, he said, was rooted not just in the strict separation of the races but "in holding Blacks down to very much lower standards" in education, housing, and medical care.[12]

While the Black middle classes tended to reside in areas like Smithfield and Enon Ridge to the west and northwest of downtown, the majority of African Americans lived in slums in North Birmingham and Southside. The latter, starting just a few blocks below the central business district, was over 80 percent African American. Its racial and demographic profile reflected the success of city leaders in perpetuating segregation through zoning laws. Reports of the Jefferson County Department of Health routinely described Southside as among the most blighted areas of the city, symbolized by its aging, ramshackle houses, which were overcrowded and lacking in central heat and private baths.[13]

PIERCE S. MOTEN AND THE SOUTHSIDE CLINIC

Born in Texas into a family of nine children, Pierce S. Moten attended Tuskegee Institute, where he helped pay his tuition by working in the office of the school physician. After graduating, he began premedical study under George Washington Carver and Harvard-educated Roscoe Conklin Bruce, head of the academic department. Later, Moten left for Montgomery to work at Hale Infirmary under the Black physician Alfred C. Dungee; he then enrolled in Meharry, finishing in 1906. Moten practiced for several years in Florida before moving to Birmingham, where he opened an office on South 17th Street.

A member of the Knights of Pythias, Moten soon won appointment as medical director of its women's auxiliary, which asked him to oversee construction of a hospital as part of the Tuggle Institute, named after its founder, Carrie A. Tuggle, known as the protector of Black orphans in the city. Moten agreed to serve as superintendent of the school's thirty-two-bed hospital. In a brief autobiography published in the *JNMA* in 1961, he noted without explanation that the hospital closed after the Knights of Pythias became involved in a lawsuit.[14]

Despite this failed effort, Moten decided to try again to address the health-care crisis of the Black community after witnessing a disturbing scene on the sidewalk outside Hillman Hospital. He later described the episode in a short autobiography: "During the depression years of 1929–33 it was common for expectant colored mothers going to the County hospital to find it overcrowded, thus making it necessary for them to return home. In many instances before they could leave the hospital grounds, the baby would be born. I witnessed a case where a Negro mother gave birth to a child on the sidewalk. The incident was witnessed by many spectators of both races which included all age levels. Men made up a large segment of the crowd (mostly colored), but not a single one offered to help (including myself)."[15]

Ashamed of his inaction, Moten began enlisting the aid of Black churches, clubs, fraternal orders, and businesses in order to create an emergency station for expectant mothers. Working with four other Black physicians in the city, "along with 25 ordinary citizens, cooks and washerwomen," he finished the task in thirty days. With approval from the Jefferson County Department of Health and Hillman Hospital, the emergency station opened in February 1932 in a small rented house at 32nd Street and 6th Avenue South.[16]

During its first few months, Black doctors on the site performed forty-two deliveries with no infant or maternal deaths, a fact that Moten attributed to the willingness of Hillman Hospital to accept the most critical cases. Because treatment at the emergency station was free, hundreds of men, women, and children began lining up to consult a doctor for assorted injuries and illnesses, which led Moten to rent a larger eight-room house on 4th Avenue South. The new facility, now known as the Southside Clinic, received donations of beds, linen, surgical instruments, and furniture from a handful of Black and white doctors in town, as well as from ACIPCO, the world's largest manufacturer of cast-iron culvert pipes. With more space, the clinic added gynecology and pediatrics to its services and began to offer prenatal and postnatal care.

During its first year, the Southside Clinic was barely able to patch together a budget of $3,000, the most that small donors could afford. After several years of makeshift operations, Moten launched a campaign to build a larger hospital. Black middle-class leaders backed the effort, including editors Oscar W. Adams of the *Birmingham Reporter* and Robert Durr of *The Weekly Review*. Prominent Black pastors joined in, along with a number of white ministers, among them James E. Dillard, pastor of the Southside Baptist Church and head of the Alabama affiliate of the Commission on Interracial Cooperation. White business leaders, like the medical community, remained largely aloof.[17]

In the end, Dr. Moten was able to raise sufficient funds to buy land for a hospital but not enough for a building. Then, in 1942, the ongoing Depression forced the closing of the Southside Clinic. Nevertheless, Moten could claim credit for having alerted leaders of the Rosenwald Foundation to the worsening health-care emergency facing the city's African Americans. In 1937, he invited its president to speak during the Southside Clinic's annual homecoming celebrations; afterward, the director of the foundation's Negro Health Division, M. O. Bousfield, requested a follow-up visit. This convinced him of the urgency of the problem, thus "setting the stage," in Moten's words, for an important breakthrough in health care for the city's African Americans.

THE SLOSSFIELD HEALTH CENTER

The Slossfield area of North Birmingham during the 1930s was not a good place to call home. The district's fifty thousand African Americans accounted for nearly 50 percent of the city's Black infant mortality, stillbirths, and tuberculosis deaths.[18] Initial efforts to address these problems came from ACIPCO president W. D. Moore; seeking to advance the Christian ideals of the company's founder, Moore sponsored numerous segregated projects on the company's 250-acre site, from baseball teams to YMCAs. Later, he broadened his vision to include health and recreation centers, securing a promise of assistance from the state and county boards of health. He also persuaded the federal government to put up $200,000 toward the cost, mainly through such New Deal agencies as the WPA and the National Youth Administration (NYA), plus the Children's Bureau. The Rosenwald Foundation agreed to cover the costs of constructing and equipping the health center itself.[19]

Built by the WPA in art deco style between 1936 and 1939, the Slossfield

Community Center started out with a kindergarten, a library, and youth and adult classes. So impressive were its activities that in a contest sponsored by International Harvester at the 1940 American Negro Exposition in Chicago, it was named the most outstanding Black community center in the United States. By then, four buildings were in operation: administration, education, medical, and recreation. The health center in the medical building was headed by a Black veteran of World War I named Walter H. Maddux, who had done postgraduate training in pediatrics at the University of Chicago. During the early 1930s, he joined the Children's Bureau, where he traveled throughout the South offering maternal and child welfare clinics.

The health center soon added a maternity service of ten beds and began offering two weekly clinics for prenatal care. At the height of its operations, the center also sponsored three weekly clinics devoted to pediatric care, six to dental problems, two to diagnoses of tuberculosis, and one to treatment of the disease. Two weekly clinics were aimed at diagnosing gonorrhea and syphilis, while two others provided treatment. For the latter, doctors followed a schedule established by the Alabama State Board of Health that involved ten arsenical and ten bismuth injections. All these services fell under the control of the Jefferson County Board of Health and four part-time white doctors known as senior consultants who specialized in one of four fields: obstetrics, pediatrics, venereal disease, and tuberculosis. Assisting the consultant in obstetrics was a Black junior consultant who oversaw home deliveries performed by Black physicians who were enrolled in training. Rounding out the staff were six Black public health nurses, one Black dentist, and one white supervisory nurse.[20]

Besides being able to treat their own patients at the Slossfield Health Center, the city's Black doctors had an opportunity to acquire needed postgraduate training. Although the Jefferson County Board of Health failed to preserve any record of their achievements, twelve Black doctors are known to have completed the program in obstetrics and eight doctors, the program in pediatrics.[21] A sampling of fifteen of these practitioners shows the degree to which they were embedded in the lives of their communities. Ten, for example, lived in North Birmingham or in the predominantly Black regions of the northeast and northwest, many of which were zoned for heavy industry. Ten also maintained offices in the industrial districts.[22]

The opening of the health center marked an immediate improvement in the lives of local residents. During its first year, Black medical personnel dealt with 803 maternity cases, which accounted for 3,129 patient visits to the weekly clinics. Of the 803 cases, 554 were for prenatal care, 175 for postnatal, and 74 for syphilis. By the end of 1940, Slossfield clinicians (as the Black doctors in training were called) had delivered 220 babies, of which 120 were done at home. There were no infant deaths (though five of the babies died within a week), and just nine stillbirths. In 1942, the *ACIPCO News* reported that not a single death in childbirth had occurred at Slossfield: "This is a remarkable record when compared with the state maternity mortality rate among Negroes, which is 89 per 1,000 against 37.7 for white births."[23]

Home visits by Slossfield doctors and nurses averaged around ten a day. Except for cases involving complications, all deliveries, whether at home or at the health center, were done by a Black physician assisted by a Black nurse, with the Black junior consultant present. In addition, Slossfield's doctors treated 1,544 sick children; of this number, 155 received smallpox vaccinations and 396, diphtheria antitoxin. Figure 4.2 compares infant, neonatal, and maternal death rates, along with stillbirths, in the Slossfield Maternity Service, in the adjoining district, and in the city as a whole.

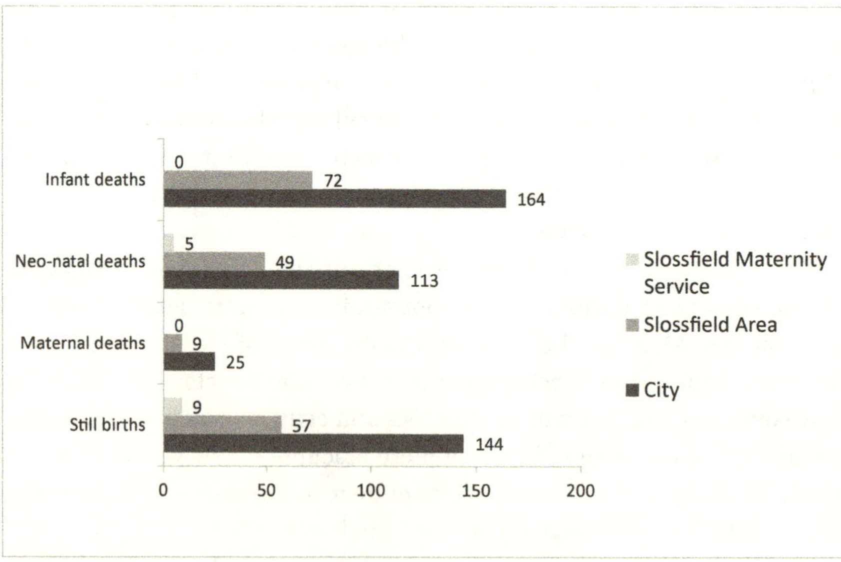

Figure 4.2. African American infant and neonatal mortality, maternal mortality, and stillbirths for Birmingham, Slossfield District, and Slossfield Maternity Service, 1940. (Slossfield Health Center, 1940, UAB Archives, MC53, 4.7.)

Direction of the clinics for venereal disease and tuberculosis remained in the hands of white specialists. In the twice-weekly clinics for venereal disease held in 1940, doctors examined 1,736 patients (involving 9,849 visits), the vast majority for syphilis, of which 533 patients returned to the center for treatment. That same year, almost 1,300 patients were examined in the tuberculosis clinics, some 400 people receiving pneumothorax therapy, which involved collapsing the afflicted lung in order to allow it time to rest and heal.

In October 1940, Dr. Maddux reported to the American Public Health Association that the Slossfield Health Center had become an integral part of Birmingham's Black community and that its twenty-one clinical periods were attracting almost five hundred people a week. Of twenty-nine Black employees, eight were local doctors doing postgraduate work in obstetrics and pediatrics: they were paid two dollars for each clinical session they conducted and ten dollars for each delivery, if followed by postnatal care. Black doctors in training could also refer their poorest patients to Slossfield when the time came for delivery.[24]

While the county health officer, Judson D. Dowling, was supportive of the center, his retirement in the fall of 1941 opened the way for department employee George A. Denison to assume the post. His attitude toward the city's Black doctors had always been patronizing: three years after assuming his new position, he wrote to Roy R. Kracke, dean of the newly created Medical College of Alabama, giving lip service to the building of a Black hospital at the college where Black doctors could practice, but adding, "I am also convinced that they do not now have the training to properly utilize such a facility and that close supervision will be necessary, both in management of the hospital and in treatment of patients."[25]

In February 1942, Maddux resigned as medical director. Fortunately, the white obstetrician who directed the maternity clinic, Thomas M. Boulware, helped ensure that the center keep its focus on maternal and child welfare. Born in Missouri, Boulware had trained at Washington University in St. Louis and completed a residency in OBGYN at Vanderbilt. In Birmingham, he worked as part of a specialist group known as the Norwood Clinic, modeled on the Mayo Clinic in Minnesota.

Boulware had two great passions in life, the first being a reduction of Alabama's high infant mortality rates, both Black and white. Of particular concern to him were postpartum infections and toxemia of pregnancy (also known as *preeclampsia*), a condition of severe hypertension after twenty weeks of pregnancy, which had to be monitored and treated early in order to increase the baby's chances for survival.

The second was charity work on behalf of impoverished African Americans. An example occurred in the late 1930s when he won a $50,000 grant from the Children's Bureau to establish a maternity service in Lowndes County, 85 percent Black and one of the poorest places in the United States. Indifferent to the fact that maternal and infant mortality rates in Lowndes County were the highest in Alabama, the president of MASA used his influence to cancel the project, informing Boulware that he could not support such a service "because that is socialized medicine."[26]

For his junior consultant at Slossfield, Boulware settled on a recent Meharry graduate named Robert C. Stewart. Born in Louisiana, Stewart had lived a more privileged life than many of his Black colleagues, a fact that his son later attributed to his father's light skin and middle-class status, symbolized by his two-lot house and swimming pool in North Titusville.[27] Boulware saw potential in Stewart and began training him in obstetrics at Carraway Hospital, ignoring its strict segregationist policies.

At Slossfield, Boulware gave Stewart increasing responsibilities, later describing him as "my prized junior consultant" and the real "workhorse" of obstetrical teaching there. In later years, Boulware was able to convince the Children's Bureau to give Stewart $400 a month in order to take a fellowship in OBGYN at City Hospital No. 2 in St. Louis. "That prepared him for his American Board examination," Boulware said, "and he became the first nonwhite doctor in Alabama to be board certified by the Board of Obstetrics/Gynecology."[28]

In a 1943 article written by Boulware, Stewart, and Elizabeth LaForge, director of Child Hygiene and Public Health Nursing of the county board of health, the authors reported that about a third of the women seeking prenatal care at Slossfield were unmarried and that a fourth had tested positive for syphilis, mostly in its early stages. The center's Black physicians had been able to treat the disease while ensuring that the women received prenatal and postnatal care. As a result, maternal and infant death rates in the surrounding neighborhoods plummeted. Between 1940 and 1943, there were no maternal deaths, and infant deaths had fallen from 23.7 per 1,000 to 10.4. Excluding miscarriages, the number of stillbirths had dropped from 42.7 per 1,000 births to 26.9. These results, the authors said, proved that high death rates were rooted in practitioner ignorance and "a lack of opportunity and facilities to provide adequate maternity care to those who need it most."

The authors stressed that as a result of their advanced training, Birmingham's Black doctors now provided to their private patients standards of medical care that were "unquestionably far superior to those practiced before the advent of Slossfield."[29] These conclusions found confirmation in a report of the Jefferson County Board of Health showing that during the years 1940–1944, health conditions in the Slossfield area had improved over Jefferson County rates by around 50 percent in cases of stillbirths and neonatal deaths and 74 percent in the cases of maternal deaths.[30]

Historian Jennifer Nelson has shown that over time Slossfield changed its community-based approach to public health to a physician-centered one focused on maternity services. As a result, Slossfield's nonmedical activities declined, and the center became mostly a maternity hospital that provided a place for the city's Black doctors to treat their private patients as well as those from the indigent population.[31] In 1944, there were 1,370 maternity clinics conducted by Black doctors at the health center, 388 deliveries, 381 live births, and 6,293 home visits. By then, 97 percent of the deliveries occurred at the health center, home deliveries having all but disappeared.[32]

With an impending loss of money from ACIPCO and the WPA after World War II, even Slossfield's function as a maternity hospital found itself in jeopardy. Although the Children's Bureau was willing to continue its support, Denison and his colleagues at the Jefferson County Board of Health showed little interest in finding local financial sources to supplant what was being lost. Ignoring Slossfield's benefits, they justified their indifference by claiming that most of the city's Black doctors had already obtained obstetrical training there. The final blow was Denison's failure to meet the deadline for applying to the Children's Bureau for continued funding.[33]

By September 1948, the Slossfield Health Center started to close down. The Mineral District Medical Society protested the closing as the loss of the only hospital available to the county's 210,000 Black residents. A letter to the *Birmingham News* written by two of the city's youngest Black doctors—Lionel F. Swan, president of the society, and Ransey G. Cole, its secretary—signaled the kinds of conditions that Black people faced. They noted that while some white doctors were willing to accept Black patients, most subjected them to segregated waiting rooms and other demeaning forms of treatment, such as calling younger males "boy" and older patients "Uncle" and "Aunt." As for the cramped spaces reserved for Black patients in white hospitals, the doctors asked, "Can any reader who has visited some of these basement wards, with entrances in a back alley, honestly say that he would not resent being forced to have himself or his loved ones treated in this environment?"[34]

Nevertheless, neither city officials nor members of the Jefferson County Medical Society acted to preserve the center. The explanation appearing in MASA's *Transactions* the following year noted that while the project had value, "it was not possible to operate without trained personnel, and the funds generated by the US Children's Bureau were not sufficient, without additional local aid, to finance the program further." In a condescending aside, the report ignored the contributions made by the Black doctors and nurses who had conducted the maternity clinics. Instead, Slossfield's successes were due to the "qualified" white obstetricians and pediatricians who oversaw the clinic and to "the fine quality of nursing supervision given by the county health department."[35]

EXCLUSION OF BLACK DOCTORS FROM THE UNIVERSITY MEDICAL CENTER

As the Slossfield Health Center began closing, another drama was unfolding that would further damage prospects for the city's Black doctors. A new four-year school, operating as part of the University of Alabama and known as the Medical College of Alabama, had opened in the city in 1945, bringing with it the two-year program in the basic medical sciences that had been offered at the university's location in Tuscaloosa since 1920. Creation of the University Medical Center soon followed and was accompanied by a series of real estate purchases in downtown Birmingham for the purposes of building new schools and specialty clinics. They included a teaching facility known as University Hospital, which started off in the now-merged Jefferson and Hillman Hospitals, both donated by the county. Roy R. Kracke, a University of Alabama graduate who had built a distinguished career in hematology, assumed the post of dean. An ambitious and skillful administrator, Kracke set about navigating the minefields of Alabama politics in order to expand the school into a national center for teaching and medical research.[36]

Wary lest they be excluded from the benefits of the new Medical College, leaders of the Black community created the Negro Hospital Association (NHA) in order to make their voices heard. Led by Benjamin J. Shaw, bishop of the AME Zion Church, the new group included numerous Black ministers and professional men, including the dentist Ernest W. Taggart and the physicians Hampton Brewer and Samuel F. Harris. Their goal was creation of a one-hundred-bed hospital, for which they would need an estimated $300,000. By

September 1944, they had only $32,000, most of it the residue of Dr. Moten's earlier hospital drive and now invested in war bonds.[37]

There were three white doctors on the NHA's advisory board, of which the most influential was George A. Denison. Writing to Dean Kracke in August 1944, Denison stressed that he wanted Black leaders of the NHA to understand "the pertinent facts" surrounding the new medical school and the possible building of a Black hospital there: "Primarily the facility is needed for teaching purposes and as such I would not be in favor of its location anywhere except in the [University] Medical Center." In other words, Black people were to provide clinical material, which may explain Denison's offhand complaint to Kracke regarding the attitudes of the Black people he was advising: "At the present time they are somewhat undetermined about location, and, as usual, a little suspicious about anything a white man suggests."[38]

In fact, Black doctors in the Mineral District Medical Society were more than a little suspicious, sensing that any plans for what was included in the University Medical Center would, as usual, end up excluding them. A resolution written by doctors Edward H. Ballard, Walter F. Brown, William L. Drake, John E. Hutchinson, Charles A. J. McPherson, Aldus S. Mitchell, and Pierce S. Moten on October 15, 1944, made clear the goals of the city's Black doctors. It demanded that the University of Alabama allocate funds to build and operate a Black hospital as part of the new medical school and that "cognizance be taken of the fact that Negroes of the State of Alabama, as taxpayers and citizens of the United States are entitled to sufficient funds to build an institution which will be a credit to the State of Alabama and comparable to any hospital built by any state of our Country." Specifically, the resolution asked that the Black hospital contain two hundred beds, the minimum needed to serve the Black population of greater Birmingham, that it accept Black physicians as staff members, that it admit Black interns and residents, and that it establish a school for Black nurses.[39]

Ignoring the resolution, Kracke wrote to the NHA in late November offering the group a half-acre site at a price of $75,000 and claiming that the sole reason for wanting the Black hospital was "for whatever service the University might be able to render to your institution." He made it clear, however, that the Black hospital would be a segregated facility: "We have no desire to own, operate, or control your facility." He concluded by mentioning the Medical College's efforts to attract a 1,500-bed Veterans Administration hospital, promising that it would be "staffed entirely by Negro personnel." Three weeks later, Bishop Shaw responded, saying that the NHA had voted to accept the invitation and that committees appointed by its board of trustees would work out the details.[40]

During subsequent talks between the NHA and its all-white advisory board, two members of the former began expressing misgivings about building the Black hospital in the Medical Center, which they feared would compromise its independence. One was the editor Oscar W. Adams, the other, Dr. Hampton Brewer. The latter was blunt and outspoken, proud of his surgical skills, and incapable of dissembling his distrust of white doctors like Denison. In December 1945, Denison wrote to Dean Kracke, complaining of the "propaganda" emanating from Adams and Brewer and asking that Kracke write to Bishop Shaw to reaffirm his promise of independence for the Black hospital, lest Shaw be swayed by these dissenting voices. Denison could not repress his disgust: "The long continued arguments among the Negroes about the Negro Hospital are sometimes provoking and, at the least, are time-consuming. I hope you will have the patience and perseverance to see this enterprise through to completion. It will take more patience and perseverance than either of us realize, no matter how well we think we know Negroes."[41]

On December 6, Kracke fired off a letter to Bishop Shaw that appeared to renege on his offer of a half-acre site in the Medical Center owing to a decision announced that same day by the Veterans Administration that it would build its own hospital there. This meant that there might not be any space for a Black hospital after all. Because Kracke was eager to lure the VA facility, which would bring enormous financial benefits to the Medical College, his expressions of regret must have struck members of the NHA as disingenuous: "I wish to tell you that if circumstances develop whereby land is not available here for the Negro Hospital, I personally, will be greatly disappointed."[42]

While there remained the possibility of finding other land for a Black hospital, Kracke told Shaw that the University of Alabama could not donate land for the building of "associated institutions." Moreover, the chances for getting financial help from the city, county, or state would "be very slim."[43] The only hope, he said, was assistance from federal sources, noting in particular the impending Hill-Burton Act, cowritten by Alabama Senator J. Lister Hill. This was a needs-based measure that combined federal grants with state and local matching funds for the construction of hospitals and medical infrastructure. Though it prohibited denial of services based on race, the new law allowed funding for so-called separate but equal facilities, a provision that the US Supreme Court would later find unconstitutional.

As for fundraising for a Black hospital in Birmingham, things seemed to be at a standstill. The banker Charles F. Zukoski Jr., who served as secretary for the NHA's executive committee, worked behind the scenes to attract support but, as he later recalled, "without much response from the white community at all."[44] As Hill-Burton money began pouring into the Medical Center downtown, members of Birmingham's Black community no doubt felt their exclusion from the city's hospitals even more keenly. In Kracke's correspondence, use of such terms as "auxiliary" and "affiliated" to describe the proposed Black hospital reveals the degree to which he and other white medical leaders relegated African Americans to the realm of the "other," not seeing them as tax-paying citizens deserving of equal medical care but as a form of special interest.

In his study of UAB, historian Tennant S. McWilliams accurately portrays Kracke as a racial moderate. Still, his ambitions at times seemed to outweigh all else. Though his political savvy and ability to attract out-of-state funds gave him leverage that most other white liberals in Alabama did not have, he was reluctant to risk offending diehard segregationists within the medical community. An example was Kracke's timid response to white doctors who opposed a plan that he thought would address the medical needs of Birmingham's Black population. It was to turn the fourteenth floor of Jefferson Hospital into a sixty-bed facility where paying and partial-paying Black patients could be cared for by Black doctors, nurses, and interns.[45]

Even this modest proposal provoked angry dissent. In Talladega, a highly respected, Harvard-trained practitioner named Arthur F. Toole penned a blistering note to Kracke, complaining that the plan would make it impossible to maintain segregation of medical libraries, pathology laboratories, and x-ray facilities:

> As I see it, this proposition will mainly benefit the negro physician who wishes to care for his private patients. The negro patient does not want for medical attention, and he may be admitted to the hospital for care by the University staff or to any other hospital in Birmingham for that matter. Now I do not wish to deny the Negro physician any recourse to hospital practice on his own. On the contrary, I feel it would go far towards improving him as a practitioner. Nevertheless, I do not feel that the University of Alabama should slip in to provide facilities for the negro doctors of Jefferson County, and I fear that it would react unfavorably toward the Medical School should the latter try to do so.[46]

Kracke wrote a fawning response to Dr. Toole, assuring him that he intended to organize the Medical College "in accordance with the wishes of the Alabama doctors. This school is here to serve the best interests of the doctors of Alabama, both present and future. We welcome any expressions of opinion on policy, as we certainly do not wish to do anything that is contrary to the best judgment of our outstanding physicians."[47]

CHILDREN'S HOME AND HOLY FAMILY HOSPITALS

Barred from postgraduate training at the Medical College's growing complex, Black physicians in the city had few options left. After the closing of the Slossfield Health Center, only two small facilities in the city, both unaccredited, were available for them to treat their patients. The first was Children's Home Hospital, located on Jasper Road in the Smithfield neighborhood west of city center. Opened back in 1922 through the efforts of Black women worried about the neglect of children in need of medical care, its original staff was composed of three African American practitioners: Arthur McKinnon Brown, Henry Clay Bryant, and Ulysses Logwood Goin. By the early 1940s, Children's Home was kept alive by fees and annual donations of $5,000 from the Community Chest. A Black newspaper described it as having four three-bed wards, plus five beds in a children's ward, noting that during the previous month it had treated thirty-one bed patients and another 120 individuals for a wide range of illnesses and accidents.[48]

The second was Holy Family Hospital, which was located in Ensley, northwest of city center, and had started off as a small maternity clinic operated by the Sisters of Charity of Nazareth, Kentucky. Despite wartime shortages, in 1943 the sisters were able to expand the facility by combining three dilapidated shotgun houses into one while using salvaged materials and plumbing fixtures. As a result, Holy Family consisted of a twelve-bed ward, kitchen, chapel, and living quarters. Though conditions were inferior to those found in white hospitals, Black doctors were eager to serve on the staff. By 1948, there were a total of twenty-two working alongside five sisters and two Black nurses. They included the surgeon Hampton Brewer, his brother Alexander Lee Brewer, Edward H. Ballard, Henry Clay Bryant, Ransey G. Cole, Henry L. Dale, William L. Drake, Samuel F. Harris, Marion G. McCall, Adolphus W. Plump, and Lionel F. Swan.[49]

The primitive conditions at Children's Home offer a poignant study of how discrimination against Black doctors affected all aspects of medical care for Black people. In addition to its work as a maternity clinic, for example,

Children's Home provided a range of medical services. Hampton Brewer and a few others performed operations there—"everybody who had nerve enough to do so," as he later put it—Brewer at one point having to operate on his own wife after she developed a tubal pregnancy.[50]

Alexander Lee Brewer long remembered his own experiences there: "When we were down to the Children's Home Hospital, Ballard, my brother, and myself used to operate together. Ballard was the anesthetist, and I was the assistant surgeon. Children's Home had only one nurse when I was here, and her name was Mrs. Berry. She ran the whole thing. Now, I don't know how much stuff she had. See, you've got to remember that in those days you had two anesthetics: you had ether, and you had spinals. We were sorta barbaric in that sense—mostly ether, applied [by drops] with the mask."[51]

A few white physicians ventured out to Children's Home as consultants, among them Boulware. "The facilities were primitive," he later said, "even the windows were not screened. It was a so-called hospital in name, but not in reality. I remember going out there and helping some of the Black doctors in obstetrics. I even remember doing a few cesarean sections out there. I hated to do it."[52]

In July 1948, the Sisters of Charity announced plans to build a sixty-bed hospital, to which they intended to allocate $60,000, with an additional $450,000 to be raised in donations. As a charity hospital for Black people, the facility would offer staff privileges to Black physicians and would be called Holy Family Hospital. Plans called for two operating rooms, two delivery rooms, a laboratory, a pharmacy, x-ray facilities, and an out-patient clinic. Though the hospital would perpetuate segregation in health services, members of the NHA and the Mineral District Medical Society hailed the effort, the former selling the land purchased for a new hospital back in the days of Dr. Moten's campaign and donating the proceeds to the drive. Doctors Hampton Brewer and Samuel F. Harris each contributed $1,000.[53]

Fundraising efforts faltered until several white business and industrial leaders took matters in hand. The result was the Negro Hospital Fund Drive, which operated out of the headquarters of the Junior Chamber of Commerce in the Hillman Hotel. The group launched its campaign in January 1950 under the co-chairmanships of Donald Comer, president of Avondale Mills, and Louis Pizitz, the department store magnate who had been an early supporter of a Black hospital. No Black physicians were named to the thirty-nine members of the sponsoring committee, though several white doctors served, including Denison. Eventually, the hospital drive managed to raise $300,000, enough to enable the Sisters of Charity to qualify for a two-to-one grant from Hill-Burton funds in the amount of $600,000. Construction of Holy Family Hospital was soon underway.

Zukoski, meanwhile, acting on behalf of the NHA, continued to press Dean Kracke on accommodations for Black doctors in the University Medical Center, believing that the Catholic hospital would not eliminate the need for a centrally located public institution to which Black doctors and their patients had access. In response, the dean insisted that the sixty beds being planned for Holy Family were "entirely adequate to service the private patients in the negro race at this time," though he did make one concession: to shift indigent and private Black patients from Jefferson to Hillman Hospital in about three years, as soon as completion of a new dental school made space available. Black doctors would then be allowed to treat their private patients there. In January 1950, Kracke again held out this promise to Zukoski.[54]

Five months later, Kracke suffered a fatal heart attack. Taking his place as acting dean was Tinsley R. Harrison, a Talladega native and head of the department of medicine. When Zukoski reminded him of his predecessor's plan to integrate Hillman Hospital, Harrison refused to consider it.[55] In letters to both Zukoski and Dr. Louis D. Green, now secretary of the Mineral District Medical Society, Harrison justified his decision by citing pressing space needs in the University Medical Center for students, medical technicians, hospital administrators, and anesthetists—in short, for everyone but Black doctors and their patients. More to the point, Harrison cited "our regulation which limits the use of the hospital to members of the Jefferson County Medical Society."[56] As he well knew, adherence to that rule would bar Black entry into the University Medical Center in view of the regulations of the society, which several years earlier had inserted the word "white" into its bylaws regarding those eligible for membership.

In the midst of these discussions occurred one of those periodic events that deflated any claims on the part of white doctors and hospital officials that the health of African Americans was a priority. It involved Lionel F. Swan, who, as seen earlier, was among those protesting the closing of the Slossfield Health Center. A native of Trinidad, Swan impressed others by his quiet dignity and soft-spoken demeanor. As a young man, he moved to New York City, where he worked as a janitor. In an interview with the *Detroit Free Press* years later, he recounted how one night a white man threw a cigarette onto a floor that he had just mopped, calling him "boy" and telling his female companion, "If I didn't do this, he wouldn't have anything to do."[57]

In early March 1951, Dr. Swan referred a patient named Emma Dangerfield for admission to Jefferson-Hillman Hospital after determining from her abdominal pains that she faced a life-threatening condition. The clerk on duty refused to admit her until $100 was paid in advance, even though one of the physicians on duty said that denying her treatment could result in her death. Mrs. Dangerfield's husband managed to get $50 along with a promise for another $50 from his employer at Southern Farmer Magazine, who called the hospital to say that the money was on the way. The clerk refused to let her in until the money arrived and a white doctor had formally admitted her. Mrs. Dangerfield was left waiting because all the beds for Black patients were taken. Frustrated and sick, she went home, where she died later that night.

In a letter to the *Birmingham News*, Swan denounced the hospital's actions. The superintendent responded that no bed had been available for Mrs. Dangerfield, claiming that there were only twenty-seven beds for private Black patients in the facility. A few days later, Swan's colleague, Louis D. Green, sent a second letter to the newspaper pointing out that Mrs. Dangerfield's was "not an isolated case, nor a situation of singling out any hospital. It is a statement of fact that is mingled and deeply intertwined in a deep-seated, generally inhuman attitude, not only of hospital admission of a patient, but the inadequacy of hospital facilities for caring for Negro patients."[58]

Reactions to Mrs. Dangerfield's death revealed a divide between the city's conservative medical leaders and several of its white civic organizations. An example was a resolution sent to Acting Dean Harrison from the Birmingham Section of the National Council of Jewish Women, saying that inferior health care for Black people "is a blot on the reputation of our community."[59] The Young Men's Business Club of Birmingham agreed, calling for space in Jefferson-Hillman Hospital where "qualified and licensed Negro physicians be permitted to treat their patients at this institution, under such circumstances as may be practicable, and with full observance of all existing State and City laws."[60]

Digging in his heels, Harrison answered with his usual litany of arguments regarding space priorities and added a new one as well: providing space for Black doctors and their patients was not part of the medical school's mission as part of the University of Alabama.[61] He insisted to a friend on the university's board of trustees that no matter how urgent the needs of Black people were, allowing community service to take precedence over education would be a "disastrous policy" that would tend to make the University Medical Center "a Birmingham institution" rather than "an Alabama institution." Far better for Black people to build their own hospital in Tuskegee, where there was more than sufficient clinical material and where white "loan faculty" could help train more Black physicians. While this would not satisfy "the national Negro group which is out to abolish segregation," it "would protect us from adverse decisions of the Supreme Court of the United States."[62]

In the end, Harrison's opposition blocked the entry of African American doctors into Jefferson-Hillman Hospital for another thirteen years. The loss of talent to the state that would otherwise have been gained by allowing Black doctors to have access to the new Medical Center's resources was symbolized shortly afterward by Swan's departure for Detroit, where he built a distinguished career and rose to the presidency of the Detroit Medical Society and eventually of the NMA. Despite the efforts of Dr. Moten and his successors, the state's medical profession had managed to beat back challenges to health-care segregation, ignoring and at times sabotaging lifesaving initiatives such as the Slossfield Health Center.

Meanwhile, the state's political and medical leaders were intensifying their efforts to secure Hill-Burton funding for the building of hospitals in Alabama. Their zealous pursuit of federal money stood in sharp contrast to their traditional antigovernment rhetoric. The irony is easy to understand. Federal assistance promised to bring economic benefits to the state while allowing it to address its health-care needs without having to raise taxes. In 1953, the state health officer, D. G. Gill, explained that Hill-Burton money was finally making it possible for Alabama to care for its sick. Since the law's passage, he said, construction had begun on thirty new general hospitals, of which twenty-four were completed, along with one tuberculosis hospital and seven public health centers. Additional applications had been filed for thirty-seven more general hospitals, which, when finished, would mean a grand total of sixty-seven, or an average of one per county.[63]

Distracted by such heady optimism, the city's medical and political elites seemed oblivious to external forces threatening their way of life in the absence of racial reforms. President Truman's desegregation of the armed forces in 1948 took place at a time of increased Black resistance to Jim Crow laws, symbolized by the NAACP's legal challenges to segregation and by Supreme Court decisions barring racially restrictive property covenants and separate law schools for African Americans. These culminated in 1954 with *Brown v. Board of Education*, which ruled that so-called separate but equal policies in education were "inherently unequal."

These milestones in the struggle for racial equality in America were greeted with hostility by large elements of Alabama's ruling classes. That included many white medical leaders whose response to external pressures for reform ranged from denying that race relations in the state were poor to offering token reforms in order to deflect criticisms of their treatment of Black patients in the hospitals. In 1950, for example, Dean Kracke and Arthur L. Bailey, superintendent of Jefferson-Hillman Hospital, described how patients were now being segregated: "Thus, one floor may be a white, pay patient floor; another a white, county patient floor; another a colored, indigent patient floor; and still another a colored, pay patient floor." The authors seemed proud of being able to maintain a segregated hospital on the basis of both race and social class: "This plan has worked out very well and we have found it quite satisfactory to hospitalize patients of all economic levels and both black and white in the same building."[64]

Such idyllic depictions clashed with reality. Nine years earlier, a writer for Robert Durr's *Weekly Review* reported that there were four hospitals in the city that featured basement wards for Black patients and that the worst of them, which was owned and operated by a major religious denomination, was entered "through an alley lined with ash and garbage cans." Once inside, the sick were forced to make their way through the hospital's laundry and boiler rooms before reaching the Black ward.[65] "South Highland, Baptist—the Black patients were in the basement under the asbestos pipes," recalled Alexander Lee Brewer. "I can remember the Black patients out at TC&I.[66] I can remember the Black patients out at South Highland, and they were in the basement over there, because I can remember visiting friends or patients over in those hospitals. You could visit your patients, but you couldn't treat them. You were just like any other visitor."[67] Dodson M. Curry remembered how the Black wards at Hillman, which in 1950 were located on the second and third floors, were crowded and lacking in minimum hygienic and medical standards. "Don't take me to Hillman," he said, was a common refrain among his patients. Herschell Lee Hamilton, who arrived in Birmingham in 1959 and later became the first Black board-certified surgeon at University Hospital, recalled his reaction when first seeing the segregated wards of two Birmingham hospitals, where Black patients lay crowded in the basement under sewer and water pipes: "I remember walking out of there the first time and asking myself, 'What did Black folks do to white folks to be treated like that?'"[68]

CATHOLIC HOSPITALS

Though defeated in their campaign for a hospital of their own, Birmingham's Black physicians had at least one consolation—the grand opening of Holy Family Hospital on January 10, 1954; fourteen Black doctors made up the medical staff, which included Robert C. Stewart, Pierce S. Moten, Aldus F. Mitchell, and eleven others, several of whom had been fighting for a Black hospital since the 1930s.[69]

The group moved quickly to fill the gap left by the closing of the Slossfield Health Center. Dr. Stewart, for example, organized an obstetrical clinic to benefit women unable to afford a private doctor; for a fee ranging between $75 and $100, expectant mothers received care for all stages of pregnancy, including hospital stay and delivery. The medical staff managed the clinic through a system of rotation and sharing of fees, and because the pay was small, the sisters charged them nothing for hospital expenses related to the clinic.[70]

Because Holy Family Hospital posed no overt challenge to segregation, white specialists made themselves available for consultations. "They didn't have to fear any criticism of any kind, simply because this patient was not at University Hospital or Brookwood," said Dr. Curry. "It was okay as long as you kept it 'over there.'" One white consultant was the obstetrician Clay Norris Wells, who one day received a call from the Sister Superior: "She asked me to be the obstetrics and gynecology consultant for Holy Family Hospital. She said my only responsibility would be to be available for consultation for Holy Family's (Black) doctors. And that when there was an OB or GYN crisis or emergency that their doctors 'couldn't handle,' then I would be able to come over at any hour I was not occupied in another hospital to the labor, delivery room or the operating room at Holy Family and 'bail the doctor out.'"[71]

The Sisters of Charity appear to have enjoyed cordial relationships with the Black staff, despite a few tensions. Dr. Curry, himself a Catholic, described his feelings toward them as "more positive than negative," remembering that they were "quite vigilant in the operating room when female patients were undergoing abdominal surgery to prevent any surgical means of birth control such as tubal ligation." One aspect of the sisters' nursing care deeply impressed Curry: "I would venture to say that Holy Family Hospital had the best [survival] rate in the state for premature children. I can attest to that because my twin boys were premature. What happened, it was so much love given to those children, and it was a challenge to [the sisters] to sit there with them at night and to see that they were fed the proper thing."[72]

For James T. Montgomery, Holy Family was a godsend. "I'm more grateful to Holy Family Hospital than to any institution," he said, "because had there been no Holy Family Hospital, there could have been no James T. Montgomery in Birmingham practicing medicine." As to the nursing staff, he said he "had very little trouble getting along with the sisters, and they almost immediately began to respect me. We often disagreed, but it was always a respectful disagreement."

Montgomery's high opinion of Holy Family was not universally shared by his patients, some of whom thought that the care provided there was inferior to that available in white hospitals. "There was never a point at which the patients would not rather have gone to a white hospital," he said, even though facilities in the Black wards at white hospitals were inferior to those at Holy Family. Montgomery ascribed this attitude to "the brainwashing that we'd undergone from slavery on up." He recalled how things changed in 1963, when he became the first Black physician to practice at University Hospital: "If the patient went to University Hospital under my care and died, it was okay; it was a just death. But all who died at [Holy Family], and there were a large number of them, [the families] were always wondering [at the time of admission], 'Will he live?' But after I could place them at University Hospital, it was a different attitude."[73]

By combining private contributions with matching Hill-Burton funds, the Catholic church was able to construct or expand three other hospitals in the state—Martin de Porres in Mobile, St. Jude in Montgomery, and Good Samaritan in Selma. There, a small number of Black physicians worked under the administrative direction of all-white religious orders, treating mostly non-Catholic Black patients. That was true even in Catholic Mobile, where an estimated 85 percent of the patients at Martin de Porres were not affiliated with the church. The hospital opened in April 1950 at a cost of $616,000, of which a third came from Hill-Burton funds.[74]

Although welcomed by Black doctors, the thirty-five beds at Martin de Porres met only a fraction of the Black community's needs. Walker B. LeFlore remembered that the facility was always crowded, with beds lining the hallways.[75] Black doctors worked directly with white doctors in the care of Black patients, but the racial divide in the city's medical community made it difficult to develop any close professional bonds. Kendal I. Foster recalled that his father, Maynard V. Foster, consulted regularly with white physicians at the hospital but maintained no kind of "amicable relationship" with them outside of it.[76]

In fact, the Mobile County Medical Society was among the most obdurate in the state on matters of race. It was also notorious for infighting. E. Chandler Bramlett Sr., administrator of Mobile Infirmary, described its leaders as a "clique," noting that during the years immediately following World War II, "they wouldn't give anybody a license to practice unless they approved of them themselves." Among those who ran the group, he said, were "a few doctors who did not go to war. And they just controlled the County Medical Society. We had a hard time getting into the society because they just blackballed us. They didn't want . . . competition." Another white veteran, the internist Samuel Eichold, described how during World War II this clique determined which of their colleagues would be drafted. The motives were pure greed: "All the doctors that they wanted out of the community were sent into the service. . . . The community became loaded with mercenaries, I would say."[77]

It is not surprising that even the most brilliant Black physicians should fare badly in such an environment. An example was Mobile native Earle Timothy Odom, a 1934 Meharry graduate who had done advanced work in cardiology at Harvard and Tufts Medical College, where he trained at hospitals in the Boston area, including Massachusetts General. He later became the first Black chair of internal medicine at Meharry. After World War II, he tried to establish a practice in Mobile, but no hospital would grant him admitting privileges. Instead, he became chief of the medical service at the TVAH, where he helped create residency programs in medicine and surgery.[78]

After passage of the Civil Rights Act of 1964, whose Title VI banned the use of federal money for any hospital that discriminated against Black people, Odom thought that the time was right to renew his request for staff privileges at a facility other than Martin de Porres, which lacked modern lifesaving equipment available elsewhere in the city. He thus left the TVAH to try his hand again at private practice in Mobile, but both Providence Hospital and Mobile Infirmary turned him down—all this despite the fact, as Eichold later noted, that Odom was a board-certified physician whose inability to work in the hospitals adversely affected health-care delivery in Mobile. Alma Foster, wife of the Black physician Maynard V. Foster, later remarked that the experience left Odom with a lingering bitterness. Whether it was this rejection, or whether health and finances played a role, as the police suggested, Odom's life ended tragically on December 23, 1977, when he shot himself at his residence.[79]

In Montgomery, St. Jude Hospital sat on a forty-acre site known as the City of St. Jude, which included a church and school. Opened in 1951 with the help of $500,000 in Hill-Burton funds, the three-story hospital, operated by the Vincentian Sisters of Charity, contained 165 beds and, like Martin de Porres in Mobile, banned racial discrimination. Until then, Black doctors had been limited in their practices to Hale Infirmary and were compelled to surrender any patient requiring urgent attention to white physicians on the staffs of segregated hospitals. Among the largest was St. Margaret's, operated by the Daughters of Charity of St. Vincent de Paul, whose Black patients were relegated to an annex.

When St. Jude opened, there were only seven Black doctors in the city, a number that had remained fairly constant since the early years of the century. During the 1950s, a small cadre of talented Black practitioners began arriving, several of them military veterans less inclined than those of an earlier era to tolerate discriminatory treatment. Along with Underwood, Wilson, and the surgeons Pryor and Winston was a Meharry graduate named James E. Caple, who had just completed a residency in internal medicine at the TVAH. Caple had served as a medical officer in the Korean War, earning a Bronze Star for evacuating wounded soldiers under fire and the Order of Military Medical Merit award for creating a safe water supply for the troops.[80]

The newcomers duly applied for admission to one or more white hospitals, including St. Margaret's. All were turned down. "St. Jude was an adequate hospital," Winston explained, "but we were interested in a little more than that. When we got here, we knew we had credentials as good or better than most people. We felt that we were as qualified as any surgeon here, and yet we were denied hospital staff privileges."[81]

Underwood felt both rejection and betrayal. He recalled that while finishing his training at the TVAH, he had talked with several members of the Montgomery County Medical Society who had assured him that the reason no Black doctors had been admitted was that none had the proper qualifications: "So I saw to it that I had as much training or more than any internist in this town. When I came back, I found out that they had lied to me. There were well-trained [Black] physicians here that had not been allowed to join the society or to get staff privileges either. Every time it came to a vote, I was turned down." One day, a prominent white surgeon, a native New Englander and a person he had considered a friend, said to him: "Jeff, I think you're an outstanding physician, and I would really like to refer some of my white patients to you. But you just don't know; if I did that, [the other white doctors] wouldn't refer patients to me any longer."[82]

Not content with excluding them from the county medical society, white doctors imposed a steady stream of petty humiliations on their Black counterparts. Underwood got his first taste soon after he opened his practice: "The county medical society ran a free clinic over on Jeff Davis Avenue, which is in the Black section of town. It was just a little shotgun house, and they gave out free samples, and they would see patients that would come there. So I tried to volunteer—these were mostly Black patients that they were seeing—and they turned me down. I couldn't even volunteer because they said you had to be a member of the county medical society to volunteer to wait on these people." On another occasion, Underwood received a notice from the society inviting him to attended a lecture at the Whitley Hotel by the cardiologist Paul Dudley White, only to be told later that the invitation had been sent by mistake. Underwood refused to back down and was finally permitted to attend, content to ignore the stares of audience members.[83]

In Selma, fifty miles to the west, Good Samaritan Hospital, known locally as "Good Sam," offered medical care to African Americans from a six-county region. Its origins dated to the early 1920s, when a group of white doctors, having built Selma Baptist Hospital, created a separate facility as a token to segregationist doctrines. In 1937, a Catholic order known as the Edmundite Southern Missions purchased Good Samaritan and asked the Sisters of St. Joseph of Rochester, New York, to help out. Though the facility at first lacked laundry facilities and hot water tanks, with only wood and coal fireplaces for heat, the sisters modernized the structure and oversaw construction of brick wings in 1947 and 1957. Thanks to an infusion of Hill-Burton funds—$94,883 in 1956 and another $664,000 in 1962—Good Samaritan became a four-story hospital with 111 beds.

Here, the sisters cared for Black victims of neglect, from emaciated children suffering from malnutrition or burns from open fireplaces to adults injured in police beatings. Historian Barbra Mann Wall has described how the sisters moved beyond their original conversion mission toward an identification with the Black people to whom they ministered. This was a matter of concern to the church's male hierarchy, not to mention Selma's white residents. While the sisters at "Good Sam" had to tread with caution, they were not afraid to embrace the communities they served. They called themselves "the New Nuns," a description they earned from their willingness to serve a mission of social justice.[84]

In 1960 white doctors held all but two of the twenty-two staff appointments at Good Samaritan, though African Americans constituted half the local population. The low number of Black doctors is not surprising. Between 1890 and 1970, only ten had been willing to brave the town's racial climate. The three still practicing during the 1950s and 1960s were William Burwell Dinkins, nephew of Dr. Pauline E. Dinkins; Edward A. Maddox Jr., a New Jersey native who finished Meharry in 1948; and Nathaniel D. Walker, a Leonard graduate of 1913.[85]

In his book *Black in Selma*, attorney J. L. Chestnut Jr. notes that most of

Selma's Black doctors "had a terrible time and either left or ended up in some awful condition." As examples, he cites Maddox and Dinkins, the former of whom suffered from alcoholism ("Dr. Maddox drank himself to death, almost literally"), and the latter from trouble with state medical authorities over his prescription practices, which landed him in prison. The accusations focused on prescriptions Dinkins wrote between August 1964 and February 1966—that is, during the height of Selma's civil rights protests in which Dr. Dinkins had tended to the injured.[86]

Although Catholic hospitals offered needed health care to thousands of African Americans, they remained limited in their impact. By the mid-1960s, the four in question had a combined total of just 317 beds, and even these remained inaccessible to patients in many rural areas. Nevertheless, for the first time, Black doctors were able to practice in well-equipped facilities, which also provided them with a network of white consultants who knew their qualifications, a small number of whom would later prove willing to support their entry into county medical societies.

CHAPTER FIVE

Civil Rights, Professional Rights

In 1947, on the occasion of the AMA's one hundredth anniversary, the distinguished Black surgeon Charles R. Drew of Howard University delivered a stinging rebuke to the organization. In a letter to its journal, he dismissed its oft-repeated arguments that Black doctors could attain AMA membership: "You and I know that it is utterly impossible for a Negro physician to become a member of a county medical society in the South. The American Medical Association has stood by the bylaws which made this so as though God himself had written the bylaws."

Drew urged the AMA to consider qualifications based on recommendations from existing Black medical societies in Alabama, Mississippi, Louisiana, Georgia, and other Southern states, where Black doctors suffered an "unwarranted stigma" from being excluded from the organization. Such treatment prevented them from having professional contacts, postgraduate education, and the intellectual stimulation provided by attendance at meetings. But even more was at stake: "Approximately twice as many Negro mothers die in childbirth as the mothers of the nation as a whole. Approximately twice as many children die in the early hours of life. The average Negro has a life span ten years less than the average American citizen of other racial origin. Yet the physicians who take care of these patients for the most part in those areas of the country where the conditions are worse are studiously eliminated from those associations and contacts which would make their job easier and their care of patients better."[1]

Drew's words acted as a call to action for the South's Black doctors, including those in Alabama. In addition to his personal ties with individuals such as Tuskegee's John Franklin Hume, who studied surgery with him at Howard,

Drew had long been active in Tuskegee's programs for postgraduate medical education. In fact, it was while driving to Tuskegee to attend the John A. Andrew Clinical Society in April 1950 that he was killed in an automobile accident in rural Alamance County North Carolina. Despite frantic efforts to save his life by the white surgeons on duty, a rumor soon spread among some Black people that Drew had been denied treatment because of his race. Though a myth, the story took on a life of its own, coming to symbolize the exclusion of African Americans from the benefits of modern medical care, which included numerous instances in which those suffering from emergency conditions were denied entry into white hospitals.[2]

Drew's life and death resonated among Black people for another reason—his pioneering work on blood plasma collection and storage during World War II, which saved thousands of Allied lives. The contrast between Drew's contributions to victory and the continued ill-treatment of Black soldiers in America's segregated army repeated a familiar theme for those who had fought in America's wars, only to be denied freedom at home.

It had not started out that way. Around 179,000 African Americans served in the Union army during the Civil War, and when war broke out with Spain in 1898, many again joined the ranks. In Alabama, the surgeon Arthur McKinnon Brown took a personal role in efforts to form a Black volunteer company in Birmingham, but things fell apart when potential recruits learned that officials in Washington had decreed that Black units had to be commanded by white officers. Leaders of the Birmingham unit refused. In the end, the African Americans who fought in Cuba—three thousand among sixteen thousand in all—were from units of the regular army who had been serving out West. Brown himself was able to join them, not as an officer but as a contract surgeon.[3]

The valor of Black regulars in Cuba made hardly a dent in the wave of white supremacist sentiment sweeping over Alabama. If anything, the sight of armed Black men in uniform infuriated white men, turning military camps into powder kegs, as happened in Anniston in November 1898. A year later, ex-Confederate general John T. Morgan, seeking a fourth term in the US Senate, told an Athens crowd that he opposed a Black man becoming a United States soldier and that if reelected, he intended to propose a law barring them from enlisting."[4]

MILITARY SERVICE AND CIVIL RIGHTS ACTIVISM

America's declaration of war on Germany in April 1917 produced another outpouring of patriotic sentiment among members of Alabama's Black medical corps who saw participation in the struggle as a way to bolster their claims to equality at home.[5] Members of the all-Black Alabama Medical, Dental and Pharmaceutical Association (AMDPA) sent a message to President Woodrow Wilson offering their services to the nation. In Montgomery, a Black dentist named William H. Watkins, who had been a sergeant in the 3rd Alabama Infantry during the war with Spain, urged creation of a Black regiment in the state: "Our people are loyal to the government and are anxious to die, if necessary, for their country."[6]

Such expressions of loyalty abounded elsewhere in the state among African Americans who were eager to discredit reports that they were sympathetic to Germany. Just one month after America entered the war, Dr. Newlyn E. Cashin, one of Decatur's best-known Black professionals, organized a rally pledging the loyalty of Morgan County's Black citizens and calling for investigations of rumors that they were heeding the entreaties of German agents to betray their country. Joining Cashin on stage were Dr. Sterrs and Cashin's father, the attorney Herschel V. Cashin. Back in 1897, President William McKinley had appointed him receiver of public monies in the US Land Office in Huntsville; the following year, Cashin helped take depositions from veterans of the all-Black 10th Cavalry, who had recently returned from Cuba and were encamped in the city. His goal was to document their contributions to victory. Now, at the Decatur rally, the elder Cashin proposed "loyalty resolutions."[7]

Thirteen individuals from among Alabama's current and future Black doctors served in the Great War, including three who were officers in the US Army Medical Corps. One was Andrew Battle McKenzie, a graduate of Tuskegee Institute who practiced in Tuscaloosa and volunteered just weeks after the war began. He ended up on the medical staff of the 365th Field Hospital, where he treated men suffering from shell shock and mustard gas and was eventually promoted to captain. Speaking before a Tuscaloosa crowd on his return home, McKenzie said that combat had stirred in him and in other Black veterans a "broader vision" that they must now fulfill. Hinting at what that mission was, another Black doctor named George A. Weaver extolled the work of the six-year-old National Association for the Advancement of Colored People (NAACP), which promised a better future for Black people.[8]

Another veteran, Elisha Henry Jones, who practiced in Talladega and volunteered a month after the war began, was assigned to the all-Black 92nd Division as a first lieutenant. By the end of the war, he was a surgeon with the rank of captain in the 349th Machine Gun Battalion, having been awarded a Victory Medal for his contributions. Arriving home to Talladega after the end of hostilities, he was lauded by a local newspaper as "the first negro doctor to volunteer [for] the war." Jones soon resumed his practice and, like McKenzie, became active in the NAACP.[9]

During World War II, twenty-seven individuals in our group are known to have served, nine of them as medical officers. They endured constant discrimination, many being restricted to support roles or assigned to the military hospital at Fort Huachuca, Arizona, home to three all-Black infantry and cavalry divisions and the largest African American military base in the country. Anniston dentist Gordon A. Rodgers Jr., who attained the rank of captain as division dental surgeon for the 92nd Infantry, spent a "humdrum" existence at Fort Huachuca: "That was during the days of the Black army and the white army, and you don't have to wonder—I was in the Black army. And most of us were at Fort Huachuca, Arizona, and anybody who was in school with you, anywhere, you could find them at Fort Huachuca, especially if you were a dental or medical officer. They didn't have Black medical officers much in places other than that."[10] Appalled by the army's segregationist treatment of its Black soldiers, Rodgers resolved to follow in his physician father's footsteps, going on to become president of the Alabama chapter of the NAACP and a leader of the civil rights movement in Anniston.

The treatment that Rodgers experienced can also be seen in the case of Jefferson Underwood Jr. Like Rodgers, Underwood would later embrace the civil rights movement, supporting the bus boycott in Montgomery while working alongside other Black doctors like James E. Caple, a decorated veteran of the Korean War. Underwood had been drafted in 1943 after completing one year at Alabama State. Following basic training, he was sent to Fort Lee, Virginia, whose commanding officer offered him a chance to take classes in basic engineering at West Virginia State College, a Black school. While expressing doubts that he could do the work, Underwood accepted the offer and performed well but, after one year, was abruptly sent back to Fort Lee, where his unit was ordered overseas: "I got ready to load on the truck, and after I got on the truck, they called me off and said that I was only a supernumerary, which meant that I would only go if somebody wasn't able to go for sickness or whatever."

Left behind, Underwood resolved to apply for officer candidate school. Fortunately, the board overseeing applications included the general who had offered him the chance to study engineering at West Virginia State. "I remember you," the general told him. "You're the fellow who said you didn't think you could make it, but I see you made it.' Underwood went on to survive the rigors of OCS and soon wore the single gold bar of a second lieutenant. In January 1945, during the Battle of the Bulge, he shipped out to Europe. Hoping to make a contribution to the war, he instead met a wall of prejudice: "I went over as an individual replacement, but I was never in anything but segregated units. My first experience with integration in the army was in France, and apparently, one of the officers in an engineering group somewhere near the front lines—it was a white unit—was killed, and they sent me up to replace him. Of course, when I got there, they found out that I was Black—this is my interpretation—but at any rate they told me that they didn't need an officer up there, and so, I'm quite sure it was because I was Black. They sent me back to another place in Bernin, France, where I stayed for a while. Later on, they put me in charge of a laundry unit that had white [enlisted men] in it."[11]

Other Black activists of the 1950s and 1960s had similar stories to tell, among them the dentist Robert W. Gilliard, who, after the war, became an NAACP leader in Mobile. In 1944, five weeks after D-day, Gilliard crossed the channel to Utah Beach, where his company was attached as a "service unit" to General George S. Patton's 4th Armored Division. In subsequent months, Gilliard served as a company clerk in a succession of combat theaters from Normandy to the Battle of the Bulge. His devotion to duty never wavered, but his view of the war remained fixed, reflecting the attitudes of other African Americans who fought for freedom knowing that it would be denied them once they came home. One memory that forever haunted Gilliard was something that happened while he was on a troop train. Picking up a magazine, he saw a photograph of a rally in support of the war on the steps of a capitol building somewhere in the South, in which the people passing out miniature American flags were told not to give them to the Black children.[12]

A Black person's prospects in the armed forces weighed on the mind of at least one member of our group who was given the option of leaving. That was Maynard V. Foster of Mobile, who had been drafted in 1943 during his sophomore year at Talladega, then sent to Fort Lee before being selected as a cadet in the flight training program of the Tuskegee Army Flying School. He completed his certification training with the 99th Squadron of the Tuskegee Airmen just as the war in Europe was ending. Given the choice of being mustered out or accepting a commission and going to the Pacific, he chose the former. "I can remember him saying he did not want to have to go fight the Japanese," his wife, Alma W. Foster, recalled. "He refused a commission so he could come back to Talladega and finish his requirements to get into Meharry." Their son, Dr. Kendal I. Foster, recalled that his father had seen some of his classmates die during flight training accidents at Tuskegee: "I think his whole viewpoint was medicine—that he wanted to participate in the war by saving lives and not taking lives."[13]

Those who fought in Korea had a different experience, owing to President Harry S. Truman's order to desegregate the armed forces in 1948. The change can be seen in the service of Birmingham's Barefield-Pendleton. After completing his degree in December 1944, the army allowed him time for a brief internship at Homer G. Phillips before attaching him to a pool of Black medical officers at Fort Huachuca, where he worked in a field hospital caring for Black infantry units in training. Shortly after the war ended in Europe, the base commander, a colonel who headed up a small group of white officers stationed there, received a telegram from Washington saying that members of the pool could be sent home. "He just couldn't believe it," Barefield-Pendleton recalled. "And I ran into a [white] major who had been in the army medical corps for three years, and they had sent him back from Europe, and he said, 'I can't understand this. How are you all getting around this? Who do you know? You must know somebody, don't you?' I said, 'I'm from Mississippi. Bilbo is my senator. You know I don't know nobody.'"[14]

Barefield-Pendleton and the other Black doctors and dentists in his unit were certain that they knew the real reasons for their being sent home: "All were Black out at Fort Huachuca. And [the colonel] didn't know it, but we got information that it was cheaper to send the medical officers around from Europe to Japan. And the other thing was if they didn't let us out of the pool, they would have to put us into these [white military] hospitals, and they didn't want to integrate us into the hospitals."[15]

On being discharged, Barefield-Pendleton opened a practice in Pascagoula, Mississippi, before being recalled to duty on the outbreak of the Korean War in 1950. There, he served as the medical officer for a light artillery unit, barely escaping with his life during the disastrous American retreat from the Yalu River that November. When he first arrived in Korea, the extent to which race relations in the army had changed became apparent: "I was the only Black officer in that group. And the outfit that I got to, I was there as their medical officer, and they were glad to see me. I mean, everybody else was white. I stayed in the medical aid station with my medical corpsmen, who were all white. My jeep driver was from Arkansas."[16]

Birmingham's Dodson M. Curry, who had convinced an army psychiatrist to rule him mentally unfit during World War II, began building a practice in his hometown until the draft finally caught up with him. Before long, he was in Korea as a medical officer with the 187th Airborne, treating far more white than Black soldiers and serving with great courage: "I [was] a combat medic. If you see in the movies where the helicopters are coming into the MASH unit, *my* unit was the one putting 'em on the helicopters. We were the battalion aid station. During World War II, they found the nearer you can get the physician to the casualties, the more lives you'll save. So they kept easing physicians up there. I was front line, and sometimes I was nearer the enemy than to the [American] riflemen. We would have to get [the wounded], and we'd evacuate 'em on choppers and send them back to the MASH units. Our job was to stabilize them so they could be transferred."[17]

EARLY FORMS OF RESISTANCE: NAACP MEMBERSHIP, THE SCOTTSBORO CASE

Military service intersected with another development in the careers of our doctors that tended to foster a spirit of social activism—their longstanding record of trying to improve the lives of their communities. While careful not to challenge segregation directly, many Black physicians sought to use their positions within the Black community to ameliorate the effects of discrimination. What Jacquelyn Dowd Hall has called "the long civil rights movement" combatted racism on multiple fronts in the decades before 1960, linking the economic and physical betterment of African Americans to the destruction of racism in all institutions.[18]

In Alabama, Black physicians served as officers of civic and fraternal orders; as board members of banks, insurance companies, and savings institutions; and as promoters of organizations dedicated to Black economic improvement, such as the National Negro Business League. During the 1920s, the list expanded to include membership in the NAACP, of which the first Alabama branch appeared in Talladega in 1913.

It took enormous courage to join the NAACP in those days. In Anniston, Dr. Gordon A. Rodgers Sr., the organization's state secretary, found that only three Black people in town were willing to have their membership cards mailed directly to their homes. Instead, he had the cards sent to him and would then distribute them. His son, the dentist Gordon A. Rodgers Jr., described his father's indifference to danger:

> [My father] tended to be an oddball. He didn't go to church. He didn't have a high praise of the preachers in town. And, I mean, that was his personality, and everybody knew that. And when they had what they called a radical topic coming up at church about what we gonna do about the Ku Klux Klan, they always asked my daddy to do something or say something.
>
> He carried a pistol all the time. All of the twenties he carried a pistol. He was aware of the fact that [when] a Black person went downtown, it wasn't unusual for a white man to push him off the sidewalk, kick at him, spit on him. But it turned out that the white man knew who it was he was picking on. He didn't just randomly pick out Black folks. When they knew they had somebody who would take it all is when that happened. So my daddy says that [you] can't die but once, and you can't live with somebody's foot in your asshole.[19]

The number of doctors in our group who are known to have been NAACP members was just twenty-three; these, plus several prominent dentists, produced a total of thirty-four individuals who can be described as medico-political activists between the 1930s and the 1960s. Though small, the group exercised significant influence over Alabama's civil rights struggles. Ten were veterans—two from World War I, six from World War II, and two from the Korean conflict. On a larger scale, of the 165 doctors in our group for whom information on community involvement is available, a total of 111, or 67 percent, showed no significant levels of civic leadership. That left fifty-four, or about a third of the known cases, whose careers exhibited moderate to high levels of social engagement, as defined above. The tendency toward activism increased over time, which can be seen by looking at the year in which the group of fifty-four earned their degrees: for those graduating from medical school before World War II, the proportion of community activists was 25.8 percent, but that rose to 53.6 percent for those who did their training after 1941. If we focus solely on the physicians who completed their degrees after 1949, the percentage stands at 60 percent. Clearly, for Black Doctors in Alabama, as for African Americans in general, the post–World War II years saw a new militancy in the fight for freedom.

These forms of community activism occurred despite the practical limitations that medical practice imposed. Dentists had more predictable schedules. Barefield-Pendleton, whose wife, Ruth, served as secretary for the committee overseeing Martin Luther King Jr.'s Birmingham campaign of 1963, saw differences in the work routines of doctors and dentists as the best explanation for why the latter were proportionately more visible in civil rights. As Dr. Barefield-Pendleton explained it, "The dentist had his patients scheduled at the same time where he could go to this three o'clock meeting or this three o'clock social, whereas the doctors at that time were more or less on standby twenty-four hours [a day]."[20]

Even more constraining was the possibility of being ostracized by the white specialists on whom one depended for referrals and consultations. That was not the only danger, as historian John Dittmer has shown in the case of neighboring Mississippi. There, economic retaliation might come in the denial of bank loans or in pressure from white business owners on Black employees to change their doctor or dentist. There was also the method of co-option, a system based on the empowerment of Black community leaders who cooperated with the power structure. Among the Black physicians practicing in Mississippi during the 1960s, Dittmer says, some viewed the youthful Black and white voting rights volunteers streaming into their communities as agitators intent on causing trouble and made it known that they would not treat them if they were injured.

Still, as historian Thomas J. Ward Jr. notes, several of Mississippi's Black physicians braved incredible dangers in the fight for civil rights, among them Gilbert Mason in Biloxi, Clinton Battle in Indianola, and Felix Dunn in Gulfport.[21] Robert D. deShazo, professor emeritus at the University of Mississippi Medical Center, says that though persecution and Klan threats had reduced the number of Black doctors in the state to just twenty-five by 1964, their ranks included some of the most visible civil rights activists between the 1940s and 1960s. Among them were T. R. M. Howard (Mound Bayou), Douglas L. Connor (Starkville), Albert B. Britton (Jackson), James Anderson (Jackson), Aaron Shirley (Vicksburg), Robert Smith (Jackson), and Helen Barnes (Greenwood and Mound Bayou).[22]

Fanning the flame of racial tensions in Alabama was the tortuous case of nine Black teenagers wrongly accused of raping two white girls on a train between Scottsboro and Huntsville in March 1931. Among their defenders was the physician Charles A. J. McPherson, who served as secretary of the NAACP's Birmingham branch. An admirer of W. E. B. Dubois, McPherson delivered regular reports to the NAACP's national office on lynchings and police brutality in the city, which he described as "deplorable and almost unbearable at times." With his help, a committee of Black citizens raised money to defend a former miner named Willie Peterson, a World War I veteran suffering from late-stage tuberculosis. In a case similar to that of the Scottsboro defendants, Peterson was charged in the killing of two white women, tried, and sentenced to death. For his efforts in defending him, McPherson received the NAACP's Madame C. J. Walker Gold Medal in 1933 for showing "exceptional loyalty, devotion and courage in the face of prejudices, handicaps and plain dangers of a southern city."[23]

Another Birmingham militant was the dentist Ernest W. Taggart, a native of rural Pickens County who had worked as a wire-draw operator for the American Steel and Wire Company in Fairfield before earning a degree in dentistry at Meharry. After becoming president of the Birmingham NAACP in 1935, Dr. Taggart took up the cause of the Scottsboro boys, which at one point included a brief flirtation with the communist-backed International Labor Defense (ILD).[24]

A few other Black doctors and dentists across the state joined in the defense of the Scottsboro boys. In the spring of 1933, Newlyn E. Cashin was one of several middle-class Black professionals in Decatur called to testify for the defense during the second trial of the defendants, which had been moved from its original venue. As evidence that the state had excluded qualified Black jurors, New York defense attorney Samuel Leibowitz selected Cashin from a list of thirty-one local Black professionals and business owners. Despite the presence of leering, unruly white spectators in the courtroom, Cashin remained calm as he confirmed that there were at least two hundred Black residents in Morgan County who were qualified for jury service and had never been called.[25]

Supporting Cashin was a Black dentist and NAACP member named Frank J. Sykes, who produced the list of two hundred qualified Black jurors. Doc Sykes, as he was called, had practiced dentistry in Baltimore before returning home to Decatur to practice and had already gained fame as a pitcher in the Negro leagues, where he was known for his still-legal spitball. Now, sitting in the witness box, he projected an aura of gravitas, his smooth-flowing pitcher's form sporting a double-breasted suit and lace-up shoes. Like Cashin, Sykes remained unruffled by the pugnacious Thomas E. Knight, the state attorney general who prosecuted the case.

Following testimony by one of the alleged victims that she had fabricated the rape account, Judge James E. Horton set the conviction aside and ordered a new trial. Though the defendants would again be found guilty and face death sentences, the testimonies of both Cashin and Sykes left their mark, as seen in a US Supreme Court decision of 1935 that reversed the death sentences owing to the exclusion of Black people from the juries.

MOUNTING PRESSURES ON COUNTY MEDICAL SOCIETIES

It was not long after Drew's attack on the AMA's segregationist policies that several all-white county medical societies across the South began accepting Black doctors as members, but only on a "scientific" or "limited" basis. That meant that Black members could not vote or be present at business meetings, receptions, dinners, and dances, and could attend only the reading of scientific papers. When the Medical Society of Georgia extended an invitation for limited membership to the state's Black practitioners in 1952, the *JNMA* objected that "this kind of gesture carries its own insult." Five years later, North Carolina's influential Old North State Medical Society urged its members to reject all such offers, which would brand the Black doctor "a second-class physician."[26]

At the June 1950 meeting of the all-Black Alabama State Medical Association (ASMA), successor to the old Alabama Medical, Dental, and Pharmaceutical Association (AMDPA), delegates voted to press for admittance into the state's county medical societies, noting that membership there would provide opportunities for Black physicians to better their skills. The president for that year, Raphael E. Tisdale of Montgomery, pointed out that white doctors in Florida had already opened their ranks to Black applicants and that the Alabama Dental Association had been accepting qualified Black dentists for ten years.[27]

The question of integrating Alabama's county societies first appeared on MASA's agenda during its annual meeting in 1952. Raising the issue was Montgomery surgeon and MASA president Thomas Brannon Hubbard Sr., who presented a motion on Black membership, as he said with "fear and trepidation," and only after reminding the delegates of his Southern roots, "The fact that we, the members of the State Medical Association, must face is that, by education and by the qualifications that we ourselves have prescribed, these doctors are recognized as reputable physicians. As such, why are they not permitted to become members of the County Societies and State Association? The answer is clearly for social, not professional, reasons. If we are to settle this question on a social basis, the status quo is undoubtedly the answer. But are the County Medical Societies and the State Association social organizations?"[28]

Hubbard's proposal went nowhere, as was clear the following year when delegates approved a report from the Board of Censors, which left little room for compromise. Using the same logic employed by the AMA, the board insisted that under MASA's constitution, any graduate of a reputable medical school was "eligible for consideration" in the county societies, which alone should make the decision. As to the idea of scientific memberships for Black physicians, the board rejected the idea out of hand.[29]

Barring African American practitioners from the hospitals had a serious drawback for white doctors on their staffs: that was the volume of charity cases, great numbers of them Black, that the white doctors had to treat. Starting in the early 1950s, some hospitals began making improvised arrangements that permitted African American physicians to practice in the Black wards so long as Jim Crow norms were upheld. In Fort Worth, Texas, for example, five Black doctors were accepted to the staffs of two area hospitals; as the JNMA pointed out, however, their standing was "without official appointments," and they were forced to sit in separate chairs during scientific presentations to the staff.[30]

An example of how the system worked can be seen in the career of Huntsville physician Harold Fanning Drake. Always easygoing, Drake never challenged Alabama's racial order. The opposite was true for his wife, Geneva Drake, who exhibited a feisty independence from an early age. A 1940 graduate of Crispus Attucks High School in Indianapolis, she enrolled the following year in the nursing program at Meharry. Upon completing her degree, she signed up with the newly created Cadet Nurse Corps, which was just being organized by the PHS at nursing schools throughout the country. She was then assigned to the staff of Oak Ridge Hospital near Knoxville, part of a secret government facility where materials for the atomic bomb were being produced. She was the first Black registered nurse to work there.

Shortly after moving to Huntsville in 1948, Geneva Drake got into a confrontation with a clerk at Belk-Hudson, a downtown department store, accusing him of waiting on white customers who were behind her in line. Worse still was an encounter on a lonely stretch of Alabama highway, when she and her husband were driving to a state medical meeting and had to stop for gas. She used the restroom intended for white customers and when she came out found the owner, who had begun pounding on the door, pointing a .22 rifle at her head.

One of Geneva Drake's most depressing experiences was her brief employment at Huntsville Hospital: "I was over there two days, two nights in the colored wing—the annex. Now the annex, they had one room that was set up for surgery. So if there was an accident—*on this table* [*slaps hand on table*]! If there was a baby born—*on this table*! If there was a surgery—*on this table*! So, I said, this can't be, because the man would come in, and he would mop, and he would go out. And I questioned it because the first night that I was over there, they had an accident [victim], and then somebody had a baby, and the only thing he did was put down some soap and water and wipe up the floor."[31]

Two years into his practice, Dr. Drake finally won approval to admit patients to the annex or colored wing. This meant that his presence was tolerated at hospital staff meetings so long as he did not try to vote or to attend any social functions. Even then, he had to avoid pitfalls. An example occurred in November 1956 when he arrived at a staff meeting bearing a letter from the newly arrived Dr. Hereford requesting staff membership on the same terms as Drake. Geneva Drake described what happened next:

> Harold could not eat dinner in the dining room with the doctors. He would have to eat in the kitchen, and then, when everything was all finished and the dishes were off, Harold could come in for the meeting.
>
> And one evening, the waiters came in and said, "Okay, Doc, everything's cleared." So Harold went in, and he sat down with Dr. Bibb and Dr. Smith. Harold sat with them because they helped him with his surgery. And there were two other doctors sitting at a table across from them, and when Harold sat down, one had a piece of pie and they had two cups of coffee, and they got up and walked out. And that hurt Harold, Lord have mercy. He came home, and he told me about it.
>
> And the next day, he was making rounds in the colored wing, and he met Dr. Grote, and Dr. Grote stopped and said, "Boy, um-um, what were you pulling last night?"
>
> And Harold didn't say anything.
>
> "Don't you do that anymore!" And blah, blah, blah. "Don't you ever do that again!"
>
> Well, I was upstairs making up the bed, and I heard the car come around the drive. He started up the steps, and he just fell up in my arms, and he cried.[32]

Dr. Hereford's membership was approved at a subsequent meeting of the staff. When he arrived for his first meeting, he found half a dozen white doctors listening to a report from the Tissues Committee, whose job was to review pathology reports to ensure that only abnormal tissues had been removed from the patient:

> The committee was asking one of the physicians—this was a respected doctor, a grandfather, second or third oldest on the staff—why he had removed a woman's womb, or uterus. This was a Black woman of childbearing age who'd been having excessive bleeding, and they were asking why he had done a hysterectomy on her since there were hormone pills and counseling and other things he could have done to stop the bleeding without having to remove the uterus.
>
> They asked him questions for ten minutes or more, grilling him in the presence of all the other doctors, and he became madder and madder and wanted them to understand why he had done the operation without his having to say it.
>
> But then he said, "I just want to tell y'all something. All of y'all have practiced here in the South. This woman was an ignorant nigger woman, and you know it ain't no ignorant nigger woman gonna take her medicine and keep her appointments like you tell her to."
>
> That stopped the discussion, and they went on to something else, and nothing more was ever said about it. It was devastating to me, as I thought first about the woman and then about how invisible I seemed sitting there, nothing more than a table or chair in the room, just a table or chair sitting there, or a fly on the wall.[33]

Across the state, Black doctors were starting to fight back. While attending a meeting of the Alabama Academy of Ophthalmology at Birmingham's Hillman Hospital, Alexander Lee Brewer heard that the organization was hosting a reception that night at The Club atop Red Mountain, which overlooked the city and catered to the city's white business and professional elites. He decided to go: "I was paying my dues, and the scientific meeting was over here, and the guys were telling me, 'We're glad to have you, and we'll see you.' Well, I didn't tell them they were going to see me that night at the social. I came home, and I told my wife, 'Now, this might be sorta embarrassing for you, and so you better stay at home." Brewer later recounted what happened:

> Being there without any close friends, I sorta meandered around the floor,

drinking my five-dollar scotch. And, of course, all the [Black] waiters, I knew they were with me, because they were looking from around the door at this Black guy drinking at The Club. I knew the boys were with me.

And finally, [one of the white physicians] from down in Tuscaloosa came up to me and said, "I don't know if they serve *negras* here."

I say, "I don't either."

Another guy came up to me and said, "I would advise you to leave." He said he was going to get the manager.

I told him, "Hell, go on and get him."

So he went and got the manager, and the manager came, and the manager was very nice in saying that he was only employed there, he didn't own the club, and would I leave.

I said, "Look here, it ain't no problem, all you got to do is ask me." So I finally got him to ask me to leave.

On the way out, I met this guy Joe Dixon[34] that I knew, and I told him, "Now, they might as well get used to it, because, hell, it's coming, and it's going to be integrated over here."[35]

MONTGOMERY, HUNTSVILLE, AND BIRMINGHAM

Starting in December 1955, the Montgomery bus boycott signaled a new stage in the fight for equality. When it began, there were only five Black doctors left in the city, three of whom were already in their seventies. The two others joined in support of the boycott. One, as noted earlier, was James E. Caple, who served on the executive committee of the Montgomery Improvement Association (MIA), which oversaw the boycott's planning and financing. The other was Moses W. Jones, a 1950 Meharry graduate and one of eighty-nine MIA leaders indicted in February 1956 for violating the state's anti-boycott law.

Though just finishing his residency in nearby Tuskegee, Dr. Underwood came home on weekends to participate in events supporting the movement. By the time he opened his practice in early 1956, he was already a member of the MIA's finance committee, working alongside his fellow practitioner Moses Jones. He recalled the mass meetings in various churches every Monday night, when Dr. King would electrify the audience: "It was a great religious experience. They would have their choirs. There would be talk of struggle, urging people to continue walking, don't ride the buses, and organizing rides for the different people to go to work. It never dawned on me that I should do anything else but get involved." To be on the safe side—and though he never told Dr. King about it—Underwood had a permit for a handgun, which he always carried with him.[36]

While thrilled at witnessing the boycott's victory in December, Underwood knew that racism still permeated the city's ruling classes, who continued to tolerate the brutal treatment of Black people by the Montgomery police. Four years later, his fears were confirmed. His wife, Olene Black Underwood, an instructor at Alabama State, was arrested while trying to help students who had engaged in a protest march on campus and whom the police were throwing into squad cars. After a long search, Underwood located the jail where she was being held, but the police ordered him to leave: "I told them I wasn't going anywhere. So they put me in jail too. And I stayed there for a few hours. They wouldn't even let me call my office to say that I was in jail and wouldn't go back." After he and his wife were released, a telegram arrived from their friend Martin Luther King Jr.: "Deeply shocked by the shameful arrest which both of you faced. However, your courage and willingness to suffer in a righteous cause reveal that going to jail is a badge of dignity and honor."[37]

Doctors Underwood and Hagalyn Seay Wilson witnessed the aftermath of even more savage acts of violence on May 21, 1961, when a white mob beat the Freedom Riders on their arrival at the city's Greyhound bus station. Wilson was at her office when she got the news. She grabbed her medical bag and rushed down to the station; her brother, an attorney who had been working with Fred Gray on civil rights cases, came along a few minutes later and spotted her there "calmly attending to the injured, clearly oblivious to her own danger. 'Are you crazy?' I hollered at her. Barely glancing up from the bloodied man on the ground, she mumbled, 'One does what one has to do.'"[38]

The following night, Dr. Underwood found himself trapped by a screaming mob of three thousand white people outside Rev. Ralph Abernathy's First Baptist Church, where Martin Luther King Jr. spoke in support of the Freedom Riders. As violence outside flared past midnight, Governor John Patterson called out the National Guard. Underwood later recalled the scene: "We were told that they were there to help protect us, but I remember at that particular meeting a woman who had fallen down the steps and had cut her leg. They wouldn't let us leave the church. So I asked if I could take the lady to the hospital to suture her leg. They told me that I couldn't, but the lady was obviously bleeding, so they arranged for me to get transportation. They allowed somebody to take me to the hospital with her. They wouldn't let me drive my car. They said you have to come back here."[39]

Despite a few acts of violence, things proved to be more peaceful in Huntsville. There, Dr. Hereford and the dentist John L. Cashin Jr. provided leadership for the sit-in campaign at downtown lunch counters launched in January 1962 by Hank Thomas, a member of the Congress of Racial Equality (CORE). Cashin, not long out of the army, saw in Huntsville's sit-in campaign a chance to make good on a vow that he and his wife, Joan Carpenter Cashin, made when first married: that they would go to Alabama and make it a better place. Militant and extremely bright, Cashin and his self-assured demeanor galled some of the white people he encountered. That included the Tennessee state trooper who stopped him one day in 1953 near Fayetteville and knocked him unconscious, possibly because he was offended by Cashin's proper English and the fact that he was driving a new Mercury convertible.[40]

Hereford and Cashin, along with a charismatic Black minister named Ezekiel Bell, were among those who formed the Community Service Committee (CSC), which plotted strategy and raised bail money for students arrested during the sit-ins. Rallying cab drivers, club owners, barbers, beauticians, and other Black workers, the two practitioners helped to plan marches and poster walks outside restaurants and theaters; they also provided bail money based on the value of their homes, as did a white pediatrician named Virgil Howie, despite the loss of referrals from white obstetricians.[41] At one of the first mass meetings called by the CSC, Hereford stood up to say that any protester who was injured would be treated by him free of charge. It was a promise he was soon called on to keep after someone poured oil of mustard on the front seat and steering wheel of Hank Thomas's automobile as it sat in a parking lot, producing excruciating pain and sending him to the Black wing of Huntsville Hospital, where Hereford had to administer morphine.

The CSC employed other strategies as well, from inviting Martin Luther King Jr. to speak at Oakwood College to picketing the Midwest and New York stock exchanges with signs urging people not to invest in segregated Huntsville. The latter was especially effective in a city heavily dependent on federal spending for the space program. The result was a peaceful outcome to the sit-in campaign. By July 1962, most merchants had agreed to desegregate their lunch counters. Just over a year later, with help from the NAACP's Legal Defense Fund and on orders of federal judge H. H. Grooms, Hereford's six-year-old son became the first Black child to be enrolled successfully in a previously all-white school in Alabama.[42]

In Birmingham, the spring of 1963 saw the beginning of protests against segregated lunch counters, department stores, restrooms, and public facilities.

Designated Project C (for confrontation), they were organized by Martin Luther King Jr., Rev. Fred Shuttlesworth, Rev. Ralph Abernathy, James Bevel, and others, and gained support from several prominent Black doctors and dentists, though some were at first hesitant to endorse the tactics used by the demonstrators.

By then, the number of Black physicians in the city stood at just twenty-seven, many of whom were getting up in years (only twelve were under the age of fifty, and eleven were already in their seventies and eighties). Still, they included several outspoken individuals, among them the surgeon Herschell Lee Hamilton, who had come to the city four years earlier and purchased the former home of Dr. Edward H. Ballard on 7th Avenue North. Hamilton had trained at Homer G. Phillips and afterward received certification from the American Board of Surgery. "This is where God sent me," he later said. "I was attracted to Birmingham like a magnet."[43]

When Bull Connor, the commissioner of public safety, used dogs and high-powered fire hoses against demonstrators at Kelly Ingram Park, Dr. Hamilton turned the Ballard House into a triage center, treating the victims and earning from his admirers the sobriquets of "Battle Surgeon" and "Dog-bite Doctor." While pleased by his support and that of James T. Montgomery, his personal physician, Rev. Shuttlesworth made no attempt to disguise his contempt for middle-class Black leaders who refused to endorse his Alabama Christian Movement for Human Rights (ACMHR), which he had founded after the banning of the NAACP in 1956.[44]

One person Shuttlesworth had in mind was the dentist John W. Nixon, a phosphate miner's son from Florida who had earned his degree at Meharry in 1951. Nixon had at first declined to associate himself with Shuttlesworth's ACMHR, but Bull Connor's tactics appear to have changed his thinking. On April 12, the same day that Shuttlesworth, King, and Abernathy were arrested during a banned march, a statement appeared in the *Birmingham News* describing the protests as "the uttered or unexpressed yearnings of every Negro in this community." The authors, most of them Black professional and business leaders, urged city leaders to create a biracial committee charged with investigating racial conflict in the city. Besides Nixon and two other Black dentists, the sixty-one signatories included the names of doctors Montgomery, Hamilton, and Alexander Lee Brewer.

Eleven days later, a "Declaration of Concern and Support" appeared in the *Birmingham Post-Herald*, voicing support for the demonstrators on behalf of the Mineral District Medical Society and the Jefferson County Dental

Study Club. The statement noted that although Birmingham had become a focal point of racial change in America, the ferment had long been present: "As members of the medical profession, our intimate contact with the Negro community persuades us that we can never again become adjusted to segregation and discrimination." The declaration was unequivocal in its praise of Martin Luther King Jr., whom it called "America's chief apostle" of nonviolence, and of Rev. Fred Shuttlesworth, whose volunteers had been left "no alternative but to present their bodies in witness." The twenty-six signatories included seventeen Black physicians and nine dentists.[45]

Though not a participant in the demonstrations, Dr. Barefield-Pendleton supported the cause in other ways. He took his turn, for example, on neighborhood watches during the bombings that occurred in the section of Sheffield known as "Dynamite Hill," which aimed to prevent African Americans from moving into formerly all-white areas. "Those were rough days," he said. "I've sat down on that corner many nights on the truck with a shotgun. And then trying to practice in the daytime." He also put up bond money for those demonstrators who were arrested.[46]

His fellow veteran of the Korean War, Dodson M. Curry, remembered one bombing in his neighborhood that was near the corner of Center Street and Sixth Avenue: "This was a hellish contraption, in that there were two bombs. The first one was of low power, enough to draw the people out. The second one was a more powerful bomb, with the nails and the bolts, and it exploded about five minutes after the first bomb." Curry, too, volunteered for the neighborhood watch: "We would put people at the intersection—one on this corner, the other one on this corner, and up at this next light—who were armed. And I would sit up. I would take Tuesday nights on sentry duty because I was off on Wednesday, and I could sleep." For protection, Dr. Curry always brought along a .357 magnum revolver.[47]

Dr. Alexander Lee Brewer was also in the thick of things: "All of this area was bombed. We used to call that 'Bomber's Hill' over there. If you look out the window, you'll see a real tall house; it's right up on top of the hill. They bombed up there. They bombed [Black attorney] Shore's house. They bombed [Black dentist] Nixon's house. They bombed [Rev.] Shuttlesworth's church out here in Collegeville. It was up on 32nd Street and 29th Avenue North. You would feel the shock wave."[48]

As the Birmingham movement unfolded, James T. Montgomery, long active in efforts to secure voting rights for African Americans and himself the target of bombing threats in 1963, decided that this was the moment to challenge racial barriers at the Jefferson County Medical Society, which for too long had stood in the way of his professional advancement. An example was his inability to attend weekly grand rounds at University Hospital, where residents presented patients of particular medical interest whose cases were then discussed. Sitting in the auditorium and hearing these discussions would have been helpful in preparing Montgomery for the board examinations in internal medicine.

Montgomery had gone to talk with Wally Frommeyer, chief of the hospital: "I asked him if I could come to grand rounds. He said, 'Do you belong to the medical society?' I wasn't at that time. He was very courteous and very nice, but no, I wish I could do that, but we can't do that. I even offered to sit in the back of the room, which I had never agreed to do voluntarily before, but the answer was just no, a very courteous no."

In 1960, Montgomery and other members of the Mineral District Medical Society agreed to apply as a group to the county medical society. He wrote up his own letter, but finding no one else ready, decided to go it alone. His first shock was the number of supporting letters he needed: "I was told that before the push with integration began in the '50s, after the Montgomery [bus boycott] and all, that the number of people who had to recommend you for membership to the Jefferson County Medical Society was two. But when I applied, the number was five."

That was not the only problem. Montgomery had assumed that the white specialists with whom he had worked at Holy Family and who knew his work firsthand would be willing to write on his behalf, but only a handful agreed to do so. "Jim," one of them said, "we want to get you and [obstetrician] Robert Stewart in the medical society, but the time is not right."

In all, Montgomery wrote to twenty white physicians. Only four agreed to write on his behalf, and it took him six more months to find the fifth person, a man named A. E. Casey: "He was head of the pathology department at the Baptist Hospitals. And when he got back—he had been in Russia for six months on a sabbatical—he called me and said, 'Jim, I have your letter here, and I'm writing a letter today.' A few months later, I got an interview with the credentials committee, and I was admitted into the medical society as the first Black in the county."

Montgomery recalled that during the two years following his admission, the society stopped holding meetings where dinner was served. After a Black newspaper mentioned his achievement, the society sent him a letter telling him that he could not "advertise" his membership. "They didn't want other people to know," he said. "They were afraid not of the Black people or the white people. They were afraid of the conservative medical doctors. In my mind, the most conservative people in Alabama have been the lawyers, and the next most conservative group has been the physicians, the group who thought they never should have opened the doors."[49]

Montgomery never looked back. A year after his historic victory, he won appointment to the staff of University Hospital, the first African American to do so. Meanwhile, he waged an unsuccess campaign for the state legislature, persuaded the dean of the medical school to support a plan for recruiting Black students, accelerated his efforts to expand Black voter rolls, and worked with white leaders to improve police relations with Black residents in the city.

Barefield-Pendleton was the second African American to win admission. One of his supporting letters was from Clay Norris Wells, the obstetrician who taught at the medical school and served as a consultant at Holy Family. Wells asked only to be able to review twenty-five hospital charts of patients that Barefield-Pendleton had treated at Holy Family: "It took me a couple of days to go through them," Wells later wrote. "In all my med school teaching I had never seen such documentation of a first-class practice of med."[50]

Within a year, the surgeon Herschell Lee Hamilton and the obstetrician Samuel Elliot Harris had been added to the society. From that point, Black representation grew slowly, standing at just five in 1969 and at seven in 1973. Still, the addition of African Americans to the group proved helpful to other Black applicants, as in the case of Dr. Curry, whose letters included two from Black physicians who were already members.

In Montgomery, the breakthrough for Black doctors came in February 1965 when Sister Catherine, administrator of St. Margaret's Hospital, decided to take matters into her own hands. She came to Dr. Underwood and said that she would ensure that he, Pryor, and Winston would join the staff. Winston, who was at the subsequent meeting where she endorsed him for staff membership, recalled that the white doctors never voted on the matter: "They'll probably tell you that, but she got up in a meeting and declared that we were on the staff." The county medical society soon voted to admit all three.[51]

Dr. Hagalyn Wilson, whose earlier rejection by the county society had only fortified her resolve to practice medicine on her own terms, knew that the actions of the white doctors and hospital administrators reflected little more than expediency. In the same month that her colleagues were being admitted to St. Margaret's, she testified before the Alabama Advisory Committee, which advised the US Commission on Civil Rights. There, she presented a blunt assessment of racial discrimination in Montgomery's medical community:

> It was I who testified before the Civil Rights Commission as to what the situation was in Montgomery at that time—the lack of privileges for Black physicians—and as a result of my testimony, St. Margaret's Hospital was *forced* to admit Black physicians to their staff. It wasn't [Sister Catherine's] convictions. They were *forced*. The government said that you own this hospital.
>
> See, the excuse was that the staff would not vote for Black staff members. You only needed one person to vote against you, and so they effectively kept Blacks off the staff. But at that time, they had the Hill-Burton Act money, which most of the hospitals needed. The government said this is your hospital. This hospital does not belong to the staff. And they were forced to integrate their staff, and so they admitted Dr. Winston, Dr. Pryor, and Dr. Underwood.[52]

SELMA AND MOBILE

Dr. William Burwell Dinkins seemed an unlikely civil rights hero. Soft-spoken and courteous, he spent much of his off-hours, according to his friend J. L. Chestnut Jr., tinkering with his short-wave radio and flying his Piper Cub while wearing helmet, goggles, and a scarf. Nevertheless, during the racial violence in the city of the 1960s, Dinkins did his duty when it mattered, a matter of no small consequence after some of the white doctors in town made it known that they would not treat injured civil rights protesters.

Dinkins did not hesitate, for example, to take on the care of young Jimmie Lee Jackson, who had been brought to Good Samaritan Hospital on the night of February 18, 1965, after being shot in the abdomen by an Alabama state trooper during a voting rights march in nearby Marion. In a 1979 interview with the makers of the documentary film *Eyes on the Prize*, Dinkins recalled having performed an exploratory laparotomy on Jackson to remove any bullet fragments and to repair internal damage. He said that Jackson had begun to improve afterward, that he was sitting up in bed and talking and was never in any real danger. That changed when hospital officials, worried over unfavorable publicity, turned the case over to a white doctor who decided that Jackson needed more surgery. Jackson died on the operating table. Dinkins, who was assisting, told the interviewers that Jackson's death was caused by excessive amounts of anesthesia and claimed that the surgeon in charge ignored Dinkins's warnings in this regard.[53]

Dinkins was again thrust into the spotlight on March 7, 1965, after state troopers and a mounted posse commanded by Sheriff Jim Clark clubbed and tear-gassed Black men and women crossing the Edmund Pettus Bridge in a planned march to Montgomery to protest Jackson's death. At Burwell Infirmary, Dinkins and his colleague Edward A. Maddox Jr. cared for the spillover from Good Samaritan, where a hundred or so injured marchers had been brought in. While they worked, the white sisters over at Good Samaritan were forcing themselves to remain silent as those white doctors who had reluctantly consented to treat the injured berated them as troublemakers while sewing them up.[54]

Two days later, Dinkins arrived at Burwell Infirmary to find a gravely injured Unitarian minister named James Reeb, who had traveled from Boston to Selma to support the cause. Around 7:30 p.m. on the night of March 9, just after Reeb and several fellow ministers had left a downtown café, a gang of white men attacked them, clubbing Reeb in the head. The diary of one of the ministers, Orloff Miller, describes Dr. Dinkins looking into Reeb's eyes and immediately calling University Hospital in Birmingham to arrange for a neurosurgeon, only to be told that he would need a $150 admission fee. Miller's diary notes that the scramble to find the fee caused a delay in getting help. In the meantime, Dinkins arranged for an ambulance to transport him to Birmingham, but Selma officials refused to provide a police escort. To make matters worse, the ambulance broke down just outside town. Once a replacement had been found, Dinkins followed in his own car for the trip to Birmingham, finally arriving at University Hospital at 11:00 p.m. By then it was too late, and Rev. Reeb died the next day.[55]

In the aftermath of Bloody Sunday, many of the state's Black doctors feared the possibility of new attacks as leaders of King's Southern Christian Leadership Conference (SCLC) began laying plans to resume the march to Montgomery. For that reason, the doctors appealed to their colleagues across the state to join the marchers in order to provide aid to anyone injured along the way. Helping in the planning was NMA president Montague Cobb; Dinkins and Maddox were to oversee matters on the Selma end, while doctors Caple and Jones would be in charge on the Montgomery end. Operating at cross-purposes with Cobb were white doctors from New York belonging to the Medical Committee for Human Rights, who described themselves as the medical wing of the civil rights movement. Its members largely ignored Alabama's Black physicians and seemed to marginalize them along the route.[56]

In the end, there were far more medical personnel than needed. With the backing of the federal courts and protection from army regulars and a federalized Alabama National Guard, events proceeded without violence, and the doctors were confined to treating sore feet, sprains, and cuts. Still, it was a historic moment for the thirty-two Black physicians from Alabama who joined the march along the way and who long remembered the triumphal atmosphere that prevailed on arriving at the City of St. Jude in Montgomery.[57]

In Mobile, the civil rights struggle saw less violence than in Birmingham and Selma, though race relations were far from harmonious. After World War I, the efforts of Black residents to reclaim the rights they had lost with the introduction of Jim Crow laws received a boost when a Black postal worker named John L. LeFlore recharted the local chapter of the NAACP. Among those who joined the chapter were doctors Escous B. Goode and James P. Dixon, who also belonged to the Non-Partisan Voters League, which LeFlore created during World War II.

Within Mobile's Black medical community, none could equal the civil rights passion of the dentist Robert W. Gilliard, whose soft-spoken demeanor masked a steely determination to combat injustice. As seen earlier, Gilliard was a World War II veteran who trained in dentistry at Meharry with the help of the GI Bill; there he met the pioneering Black dentist of Mobile, Edward T. Belsaw, who recommended the city as a promising place to start a practice. Gilliard settled there in 1950, treating mostly shipyard workers, about a fifth of whom were white. Not long after his arrival, LeFlore invited him to a meeting of the NAACP, where the new dentist announced that he was ready to join the cause. Afterward, the chapter chose him to sit on its executive board, a position he held until Alabama outlawed the organization. When the NAACP returned to the state in 1964, Gilliard became president of the local chapter.[58]

While the NAACP focused its efforts on desegregating the city's department stores and grocery chains, the battle over Black membership in the Mobile County Medical Society was starting to heat up. Eager to acquire certification of compliance with federal requirements for hospital desegregation in order to start the flow of Medicare dollars, the society granted membership to doctors Goode and Dixon and four others, who now enjoyed staff privileges at Mobile General. Three of the city's Black physicians chose not to apply for membership, which left only Maynard V. Foster and his nephew LeBaron A. Foster outside the fold.

Since 1963, Maynard V. Foster, a member of the NAACP, had been speaking out against racial discrimination at Mobile General. In meetings of the Gulf Coast Intra-Medical Society, he denounced the hospital's requirement that an applicant for staff membership had to belong to the county medical society, which required four letters of recommendation from existing members. Foster argued that obtaining such letters, even from younger members having moderate views on race, was almost impossible, so fearful were they that their colleagues would retaliate by ceasing to refer patients to them.

In preparation for a lawsuit, Foster and his nephew submitted letters of application to Mobile General, which the administrator rejected. As expected, the basis for the rejection was that they were not members of the county medical society and that their applications did not have the requisite letters of endorsement. With support from Non-Partisan Voters League and the NAACP's Legal Defense Fund, the Fosters filed suit in US District Court, alleging racial discrimination in violation of the Equal Protection Clauses of the Fourteenth Amendment and the Civil Rights Act of 1964.

In January 1967, the Fosters' lawsuit was tried in US District Court without a jury before Judge Daniel H. Thomas, a political conservative whom civil rights activists viewed as unsympathetic to their cause. True to form, Thomas ruled that the requirements for admission to the medical staff of Mobile General, including membership in the county medical society, were reasonable and that there was no evidence of racial discrimination at the hospital in that it had already admitted several Black physicians.[59] One month after Thomas's ruling, the local draft board cancelled LeBaron A. Foster's deferment status and reclassified him as 1-A, or available for military service. It is possible, though unlikely, that the timing was coincidental: Foster was already thirty years old with seven children and was one of only twelve Black doctors in a city containing over sixty-seven thousand African Americans.[60]

Maynard V. Foster pressed on, turning next to the United States Court of Appeals, Fifth Circuit. In the meantime, the Non-Partisan Voters League had submitted a petition to the Department of Health, Education, and Welfare (HEW), asking it to desegregate the city's hospitals. Of the largest, only Providence had begun making progress toward compliance with Title VI, owing largely to the efforts of a white internist named Jean Cowsert, president of the medical staff, who convinced her fellow practitioners to abandon any further resistance to desegregation. One of only two women in her class,

Cowsert finished her training at the University of Alabama Medical School in 1954 and returned to practice in her native Mobile. Her courage was notable at this juncture, but it came at a price, both in the flight of white patients from Providence to Mobile Infirmary and in the enmity her actions stirred up in the county medical society.

By the early summer of 1966, with the deadline for implementation of Medicare fast approaching, Mobile's hospitals were among 327 in the nation that remained uncertified.[61] Finally, on June 30, Providence, Mobile General, and Martin de Porres received certification; Mobile Infirmary did not, a bitter blow for a facility that had only recently completed a new wing of one hundred beds that would now remain vacant until Medicare dollars began to flow in. Still, the county medical society, in the words of the *Southern Courier*, a newspaper edited by white undergraduate writers for the *Harvard Crimson* who had come south to cover civil rights news, resolved to make "a last-ditch stand" at Mobile Infirmary, recommending that its doctors admit only white patients while referring Black patients to Providence, a tactic that LeFlore duly reported to HEW.[62]

Six months after implementation of Medicare, the US Office of Equal Health Opportunity (OEHO), which oversaw compliance for HEW, reported that white doctors at Mobile Infirmary were continuing to send Black patients elsewhere.[63] The war between OEHO and Mobile Infirmary took an even darker turn in early 1967. Dr. Cowsert, who also belonged to the staff at Mobile Infirmary, had earlier provided to OEHO the names of twenty-five doctors there who were leading the opposition to admitting Black patients, the latest in a series of confidential reports she made regarding violations of the Civil Rights Act of 1964.

On January 27, 1967, Dr. Cowsert was found dead outside her home, shot through the chest by her own .38 caliber revolver, which was discovered lying beneath her body. The disappearance of autopsy reports and police records made the circumstances more than a little suspicious, despite police claims that she had been responding to the sound of breaking glass in her kitchen window and accidentally shot herself when she stepped outside.[64] Eager to resolve the impasse, and buckling under pressure from Senators J. Lister Hill and John Sparkman and from Governor George C. Wallace, HEW finally issued a certificate of compliance for Mobile Infirmary in July, against the wishes of local OEHO officials.

There was at least good news on another front. In June 1968, the United States Court of Appeals, Fifth Circuit, reversed the finding of the lower court in the lawsuit brought by the Fosters against Mobile General. Writing for the court, Justice Homer Thornberry agreed with the lower court that hospital boards had the right to impose professional and ethical criteria in granting staff membership but concluded that Mobile General's bylaws were unrelated to such considerations: "The requirement that a doctor must be a member of a medical society in order to serve on the staff of a public hospital violates on its face the Fourteenth Amendment."

The ruling stressed that it was the sick who suffered most from this arbitrary exclusion in that the Black doctor's patients were "denied the use of the Hospital's modern electronic and mechanical equipment and emergency lifesaving devices and materials readily available in this Hospital which operates on a large scale and has access to substantial public funds."[65] Though the Fosters' victory established a precedent only within the six-state area of the Fifth Circuit, it was an important milestone in opening up hospitals to African American doctors and echoed similar court rulings against hospital boards that rejected applicants based on arbitrary bylaws.[66]

WHITE RESISTANCE TO HOSPITAL DESEGREGATION

By 1965, Black practitioners were accelerating their drive to end racial discrimination in Alabama's hospitals, but the task was not easy. In August of that year, the *Southern Courier* assailed the state's medical establishment for dragging its feet, noting that many Black doctors remained outside the fold.[67] In fact, MASA rosters the following year still showed fifty-seven Black physicians as nonmembers of their local societies. Three years later, the number stood at thirty-five. Only in 1969 did membership in MASA appear to be open to all licensed Black physicians, its rosters having by now been purged of the abbreviation "col." after their names. But problems remained. The biggest was the slow pace of hospital desegregation, which proceeded in fits and starts as administrators delayed and obfuscated, hoping to mislead federal authorities by offering token concessions.

A case in point was Anniston Memorial Hospital. Back in 1950, the facility announced that it would allow the city's three Black doctors to admit patients for deliveries and for "medical, minor surgical, and obstetrical therapy," though they were confined to the segregated ward.[68] Five years later, the hospital had begun expanding with the help of $500,000 in Hill-Burton funds and assured the government that it would not maintain segregated wards. Nevertheless, Black patients continued to be shunted off to a separate unit known as Block One, which had its own entrance and maternity ward.

In August 1964, Dr. Gordon A. Rodgers Jr. went to see a patient in the hospital, where a receptionist told him that he would have to leave the front entrance and use the side door leading to Block One. Stung by these remarks, he sought the help of Black attorney Oscar W. Adams Jr. of Birmingham, who filed suit in Federal District Court against the city of Anniston and the hospital administrator. For once, justice was swift, as Federal District Judge Seybourn H. Lynne enjoined Anniston Memorial from practicing racial discrimination. By June of the following year, the hospital administrator reported that the facility had been fully integrated.[69]

Meanwhile, the *Southern Courier* continued to accuse hospital officials of resisting desegregation, among them Birmingham's Lloyd Noland and South Highland Infirmary.[70] The US Commission on Civil Rights found others resorting to various artifices in hopes of evading the law. In Tuscaloosa, the Druid City Hospital, which funded an addition with Hill-Burton funds, began converting rooms having four beds into two beds and those having two beds into one—all to avoid placing Black and white patients together, even if it meant reducing the number of available beds.[71]

As to the reception awaiting Black physicians who joined formerly all-white hospital staffs, Dr. Montgomery's experiences were typical. While he was under no illusions as to why he was there—as he said later, the reason was the hospitals' fear of losing Medicare dollars—he found working conditions less than ideal: "I could walk in the lounge in the morning where you left your coat downstairs, and I would say, 'Good morning,' and you hear everybody's voices, [and suddenly] there was hardly a whisper. Yet I'd meet the same doctor on the floor when none of his white friends [was around], and he was open and hand-shaking and everything. They were afraid of their associates."[72]

Forgotten among the victories of the 1960s was the fate of other Black physicians left by the wayside. One was Alexander Lee Brewer, whose letters requesting an application for membership were routinely ignored by the Jefferson County Medical Society. When he finally managed to get a copy, he tried to convince five members to write on his behalf. The first he approached was a local white ophthalmologist: "He said, 'Ah, I would like to, but I tell you, I'm afraid. I'm afraid that the ones that are referring me patients will stop. And so I'm not gonna do it.' In other words, he wasn't afraid of me, he was afraid of the other white physicians blackballing him."

Next, Brewer asked a local ophthalmologist whom he had known while training in Chicago: "The first damn thing he told me [was], 'Now, you know

I don't believe in any of that [segregation], but I'm gonna ask my partner as to what I should do.' Well, as yet I haven't gotten an answer from him. I don't know whether he's dead or whether he's retired or what. But I haven't heard from him."

Brewer finally gave up trying: "It never did pick up around here. I might say that after so long, [with] the number of Black specialists coming in [today], that they now think it's relatively easy. Most of the fellows here don't realize what we went through down through the years. They never realize [the] problems with Blacks that we had. See, I was the first one here, the first Black specialist, the first [Black] ophthalmologist. I might say that we had all the knocks and bruises."[73]

CHAPTER SIX

An Unfinished Revolution

The unequivocal triumphs of science in the conquest of disease have few parallels in the social history of medicine. Though the civil rights movement brought new opportunities for Black physicians in Alabama, the struggle to achieve professional equality during the 1960s constituted an unfinished revolution for them and their patients, a fact that was not immediately grasped by the scores of young medical graduates opening practices in the state during the 1970s and 1980s.

By 1983, for example, the number of Black physicians in Birmingham was already showing evidence of a slow but steady ascent and now stood at thirty-two, up from twenty-three a decade earlier. All but three had received their training during the post-civil rights era, and five were women, the first hint of a demographic shift that would alter the profile of the state's Black medical corps over the next three decades. Within a few years, the number of Black women graduating from the nation's medical schools began to outstrip that of men, and by 2008 women accounted for two-thirds of all African American medical students. Of 511 Black physicians practicing in Alabama that year, just over half were women.[1]

The Birmingham group of 1983 typified other changes as well. Three-fourths specialized in one of four primary care fields: family or general practice, internal medicine, pediatrics, and OBGYN. The dominance of primary care fields was typical of Alabama's post-1970 Black physicians and meant that, like their predecessors, they would continue to serve on the front lines of health care. Nationally, Black doctors by 1990 included higher proportions of primary care givers than their white counterparts—50 percent for Black men and 76 percent for Black women, as opposed to 42 percent for white men and 57 percent for white women. By 2008, around 55 percent of all Black physicians in the nation served in primary care fields; in Alabama, the figure was 69 percent, the majority of them in office-based practices.[2]

New opportunities for advanced training during the post-civil rights era produced significant increases in the state's number of African Americans doctors. In 1970, their proportion relative to all doctors in the state stood at just 2.4 percent, comparable to the national figure of 2.2 percent. Over the next two decades, Alabama's percentages continued to parallel the national average but by 2000 had surpassed it. At that point, the number of Black physicians in the state had risen to 626, now constituting 7.2 percent of the state's medical corps, as compared with 4.5 percent nationally.

While a significant step forward, Alabama's proportion remained far below the percentage of Africans Americans relative to the state's population as a whole, which in 2000 stood at 26 percent. There were 47 Black doctors per one hundred thousand African Americans, a medical ratio similar to that of Arkansas (48) but inferior to that of Louisiana (58) and Georgia (82). Among the states of the former Confederacy, Alabama ranked third from the bottom, just above South Carolina and Mississippi.[3]

While part of Alabama's increase reflected the entry of women into the profession, significant numbers of both men and women benefitted from affirmative action programs. According to health-care researchers Gary King and Robert Bendel, the number of Black physicians in the United States grew by 124 percent during the 1970s, then declined to a 59 percent rate of increase during the 1980s as a result of mounting political attacks on affirmative action.

Dr. James T. Montgomery had little patience for such attacks, remembering how the system was once stacked against him and other African Americans. Years later, after being appointed to the medical school faculty, he discovered that there were no Black students in the entering class: "That's when I got them to agree, of a hundred places, save me ten places for Black kids. I wanted to get these kids admitted with the records they could bring from their colleges. They may not be at the same level going in, but they should not come out at any level less than the other people. And they agreed to do that. I interviewed every Black kid when we finally got them to agree to hold some slots open."[4]

Nationally, such efforts to give young African Americans a chance proved effective. By 1974, minority enrollment in formerly all-white medical schools had grown by 10 percent, though the pace of increase was slowed by the US

Supreme Court's *Bakke* decision four years later, which banned quotas in college admissions but retained affirmative action by allowing race to be considered in the interest of educational diversity.[5] Nevertheless, figures compiled by the AAMC show that by 2013 African Americans constituted just 5.8 percent of all medical school graduates and only 4.1 percent of all doctors practicing in the United States, at a time when the Black population stood at 13 percent. The drop in recruitment was most visible among Black men, whose numbers among applicants to medical school declined from 1,410 in 1978 to 1,337 in 2015.[6] By the latter date, Alabama had 519 African American physicians, representing 6 percent of all doctors in the state. Its proportion put the state above Arkansas (1.4 percent) but below Georgia (12.7), Mississippi (7.7), and Louisiana (6.7).

POST-1970 STATUS OF AFRICAN AMERICANS IN HOSPITALS

Opposition to affirmative action was not the only barrier to recruiting African Americans. Despite new civil rights laws, many white practitioners in Alabama persisted in their refusal to grant professional recognition to Black colleagues. It was a pattern mirrored nationally in the AMA's 1965 campaign to torpedo a proposal of HEW requiring hospitals and doctors receiving federal funds to sign an agreement not to discriminate against patients or doctors on the basis of race. A firestorm of resistance, which saw white physicians protesting that their code of ethics already banned discrimination and that a required oath was demeaning, forced HEW to back down. The result was that the medical profession was at times able to avoid compliance with civil rights laws.[7]

Few members of Alabama's Black medical corps needed reminding of where they stood. In 1979, Birmingham journalist Howell Raines described in the *New York Times* the coolness with which many of the city's hospitals responded to staff requests from Black physicians. Meharry graduate Isaac C. Ravizee, a fellow of the American College of Obstetricians and Gynecologists, recounted to Raines the evasive response he got when he applied for staff membership at Carraway Methodist Hospital, not far from where he had grown up. The hospital attorney with whom Ravizee dealt admitted to Raines that she had "some reservations because I was unsure of his motives. I was being particularly guarded, so I didn't say anything that could be misconstrued." Ravizee had a simpler explanation: "They didn't come right out and say it, but I know Birmingham. Race is the bottom line here. That comes before credentials or anything."

No one understood that truth better than Samuel W. Sullivan Jr., a board-certified OBGYN specialist who in 1970 shared honors with Richard C. Dale in being one of the first Black medical graduates of the University of Alabama. While Sullivan reminded Raines that discrimination against Black physicians was not confined to Alabama, he stressed that Birmingham had a special responsibility because of its poor history of race relations. As an indication of the continuing need to defend Black doctors, Sullivan had already agreed to serve as president of a revitalized Mineral District Medical Society, which had been dormant since the late 1960s.

Raines reported that none of the city's eighteen hospitals refused staff privileges for Black physicians outright but that they often took a long time to respond or simply ignored the doctors' applications. In some instances, administrators encouraged Black physicians to apply instead to Community Hospital, the old Holy Family. Besides Carraway, the worst offenders were the two Baptist medical centers—one at Princeton and the other at Montclair—and St. Vincent's, a Catholic facility. Patience Hodges Claybon, who in 1974 became the first Black woman to graduate from the University of Alabama School of Medicine and stayed on to complete a residency in psychiatry, recounted how she had been turned down by the Princeton Baptist Medical Center because her field there was "overcrowded," even though she was the city's only Black psychiatrist.

A board-certified cardiologist named Clifford Latting, who had completed a residency at the University of Chicago, told Raines that one white colleague at UAB had discouraged him from applying there because "he didn't feel the faculty would be positive about taking on another Black." Latting characterized the city's medical profession as being "a closed community," remarking that whenever a Black physician applied at a white-run hospital, "they always have enough of whatever you're offering."[8]

Being allowed to practice at formerly all-white hospitals in Alabama was only the start of trouble for some African Americans, as was true in other parts of the nation. As W. Michael Byrd and Linda A. Clayton have noted, Black doctors lived "constantly at tiptoe stance, never quite knowing what to expect next." Employing peer reviews in the name of quality control, white physicians in Detroit, Chicago, Houston, Fort Worth, and other cities carried out veritable purges of African American staff members. A national survey of 236 Black physicians in 1994 found 99 percent reporting that they had experienced discriminatory treatment, from peer reviews and staff promotions to Medicare and Medicaid reimbursements.[9]

The first generations of Black students who succeeded in gaining admission to formerly all-white medical schools also felt the glare of heightened scrutiny. Damon Tweedy, who trained at Duke University during the 1990s and later became a psychiatrist on the faculty, found it hard to endure the professors' endless comparisons of disease morbidity rates among white people and Black people, invariably to the detriment of the latter. His worst moment came when a professor spotted him entering the auditorium after a break and came over to ask if he was there to fix the lights. When Tweedy answered that he had nothing to do with the lights, the professor asked, "Then what are you doing here in my class?"[10]

Such experiences help to explain why Howard and Meharry retained their appeal. For Kendal I. Foster, son of Mobile's Maynard V. Foster, the choice was never in question: "I applied to Howard and Meharry, and I was accepted to both schools. I did not want to deal with the racism that I knew was institutionally inherent in [white schools]."

In Montgomery, Jefferson Underwood III, whose father helped to destroy racial barriers in the city's hospitals, felt the same way, having never forgotten the trauma of being among the first Black students to enter Bellingrath Junior High School. His worst memories came after white students learned of the death of Martin Luther King Jr., a close family friend: "I remember kids coming to school all happy and saying, 'How do you feel about Martin Luther *Coon* being killed?' But none of those kids who were joyous and showing a lot of elation knew that the year before, I was with him, or when the great March on Washington occurred and he did his 'I Have a Dream' [speech], that his kids were playing with us that same weekend." Underwood made a promise to himself that he would never go to a white school "until I had something that they cannot take away from me."[11]

Black women contemplating careers in medicine had to overcome the challenge of both race and gender. An example was Janice Morton-Hunte. After graduating as valedictorian of her class at the Alabama Lutheran Academy in Selma, where she fell in love with biology, she entered the University of Alabama. She did so "because George Wallace stood in the door and said, 'No Blacks are coming into this school,' and that sealed it for me." Deciding on medicine as a career, Morton-Hunte enrolled at the University of South Alabama College of Medicine in Mobile, which was created in 1973 as part of the ten-year-old University of South Alabama (USA). Her first reactions after arriving on campus reflected the experiences of many other young African Americans: "When I walked into the orientation for new medical students, I looked into a sea of white faces as people were talking to each other, and, you know, the din of nothing going on and people waiting. I looked over this room, and way over there, there was one other Black person, and we went to each other like we knew each other. He was as glad to see me as I was to see him. It was like, 'Oh my God, who knew there would only be white people here?'"

Although Morton-Hunte was more than capable of doing the work, some of her professors were less than helpful, like the one who misled her on what material would be covered on their next examination. On another occasion, a biochemistry instructor was openly hostile, refusing to answer a question: "He told me if I had read the chapter, I should know the answer to the question. Of course, this is in front of the whole class." With encouragement from her mother, Morton-Hunte eliminated all social activities and made medical study the focus of her life. In the process, she discovered two important sources of emotional support. One was a South American woman on the faculty at whose office she often stopped to talk. The other was the school's Black workers: "The maintenance staff at the medical building were Black, and I was on the home team. I mean, they encouraged me."[12]

LEGISLATIVE ATTACKS ON LARGE MEDICAID PROVIDERS

In no other area did the post-1970 backlash against the ascendancy of Black doctors in Alabama reveal itself more clearly than in the medical profession's hostility to programs of the Great Society. Medicare tended to be the exception owing to the fact that it was paid for by the federal government and benefitted far more elderly white people than Black people. By contrast, Medicaid was designed to help poor people of all ages and included large segments of the Black population. Moreover, it was funded by state as well as federal money, though, as a poor state, Alabama enjoyed a three-to-one federal matching rate.

When Alabama's Medicaid program started in 1970, five years after its passage by Congress (the state was one of the last to implement it), federal dollars paid 78.54 percent of its expenses. Despite this federal largess, shortfalls in the state Medicaid budget, reflecting a determination to keep tax rates low, soon spelled trouble. The subsequent reduction of services produced one of the nation's most tight-fisted programs when measured by eligibility, services, and physician payments. Where monthly payments per recipient averaged $130.38 nationally in 1976, Alabama paid just $78.74, placing it near the bottom of the states.[13]

Despite their hostility toward Medicaid, the state's medical elites exercised enormous power over its implementation. Although MASA was a private association of doctors, legislation passed back in 1875 gave it unprecedented powers, decreeing its membership to be synonymous with the State Board of Health. As one contributor to the state medical journal later remarked, MASA became in a single stroke "the State Board of Health, the State Board of Medical Licensure, the State Board of Medical Examiners. No other body of doctors anywhere carried so much authority, responsibility, and burden. Now they had the whole bundle dropped in their laps."[14]

The top-heavy, physician-rich structures that controlled the state's public-health bureaucracy ended to reinforce pressures for conformity at the top, devoid of moral vision and consistent with the social values of white male practitioners. Added to this was the unhealthy marriage between Alabama's political and medical leadership, which was rife with conflicts of interest between the health-care needs of citizens and the professional interests of doctors. Through its lobbying arm in Montgomery, MASA directed money toward candidates who favored the economic interests of the profession. For that reason, the organization could boast important friends in the legislature.

Medicaid provided still another structure for enforcing medical authority. In accordance with an agreement worked out between Alabama and the federal government, the state health officer oversaw daily operations of the program and reported to a State Committee of Public Health, whose sixteen members included twelve physicians belonging to MASA. This committee in turn answered to the State Board of Health, the only one in the nation dominated entirely by physicians.[15] This meant that the same medical men who had long decried federal activism in health care as socialism ended up controlling Medicaid's fate. As the program began encountering financial problems, even the state health officer who was charged with running the program could barely conceal his glee. He described Medicaid as having imposed "a horrendous burden" on Alabama: "I admit my bias when I note the fiasco of Medicaid, which was spawned in a welfare atmosphere without the advice, counsel, and assistance of health professionals at all levels."[16]

Most Black doctors in the state welcomed Medicaid with open arms, in contrast with white practitioners, many of whom shunned it entirely. The state was not unique in this regard; nationally, about a quarter of primary care physicians refused to treat Medicaid patients or did so only on a limited basis. A survey of 3,482 physicians in 1977 found that 21.6 percent had no Medicaid patients; another 49.2 percent had practices in which such patients accounted for just 10 to 20 percent of their caseloads. Doctors for whom Medicaid patients constituted 30 percent or more of their clienteles made up just

15.8 percent of the total. These low levels of participation meant that a small minority of doctors provided the bulk of medical care for poor people. While excessive paperwork and low fees were given as the primary reasons for opting out of the program, the fact that Black people constituted a significant portion of eligible patients also played a role. Later studies confirmed this tendency, showing the importance of race, rather than poverty alone, in helping to determine rates of Medicaid participation. In areas where the poor are nonwhite, participation levels have been historically low, and this in turn has perpetuated health-care inequalities.[17]

Though the percentage of white physicians in Alabama who participated in Medicaid cannot be determined, it appears to have been even smaller than the national surveys indicated. Dewey White Jr., a Birmingham pediatrician and member of the state senate, was unable to provide a precise figure during testimony before a subcommittee of the US House of Representatives in 1980, where he appeared in support of a bill to give Alabama more control over its Medicaid program. Dewey could say only that in counties having large numbers of people who were eligible for the program, the number of physicians appeared to be sufficient, though he added that a substantial number of doctors in Birmingham refused to accept Medicaid patients.[18]

A survey of thirty-six local physicians taken by the *Anniston Star* in 1980 found that only half accepted Medicaid patients, despite the presence of ten thousand eligible residents in the county. At the Gadsden Neighborhood Health Clinic in nearby Etowah County, a nurse practitioner observed that "the big problem here is the fact that only two doctors in Gadsden, a city of 60,000, will accept Medicaid patients, which means many low-income people cannot get medical attention. The local health department is overrun with patients and has referred some to us."[19]

The Gadsden Neighborhood Health Clinic was the work of a Black public health activist and nurse named Roberta O. Watts, who had won an HEW grant of $792,548 for creating a private, nonprofit group called the Etowah Quality of Life Council. The clinic had opened in late 1978 in a Black housing project and was the first of several in the northern and southeastern parts of the state operating under the council's auspices. The one in Gadsden featured a full-time nurse-practitioner who performed patient histories and physical examinations. James W. Stewart, a Meharry graduate who had practiced in the city since 1944, did consultations and prescribed medications. After six months, the clinic was seeing between twenty and thirty patients a day, many of them expectant mothers in their sixth or seventh month who had never seen a doctor.[20]

White doctors complained that such federal spending created a competitive disadvantage for their own practices. Their greatest anger was directed toward those practitioners who were able to build large Medicaid practices, though most of these were far from being the so-called Medicaid Mills being denounced by enemies of the program across the country. While Jefferson, Montgomery, and Mobile counties, where African Americans constituted significant percentages of the population, were among the regions with the highest number of Medicaid payments to doctors and patients, poor white inhabitants of Piedmont, the Wiregrass, the Tennessee Valley, the Appalachian northeast, and other rural areas claimed, in absolute terms, a larger portion. In 1976, white people received 61.3 percent of the state's Medicaid payments, as opposed to 38.6 percent for nonwhite people. As a proportion of their respective numbers, however, African Americans depended on the program more than white people did.

Nor were widespread fraud or excessive payments to Black providers responsible for increased pressures on the state's Medicaid budget. In 1976, payments to doctors represented only 10 percent of Medicaid expenses; a fifth went to inpatient hospital care, and almost half went to nursing home care, where costs in both Alabama and the nation had exploded. In May 1977, Dr. Richard A. Thigpen, director of the Alabama Law Institute who was then serving as acting president of the University of Alabama, reported to a legislative committee that news stories "cast unfair impressions about many of our state Medicaid providers" and that serious abuses were minimal.[21]

Thigpen was referring to the lists of the highest Medicaid earners in the state that newspapers began publishing during the 1970s. While the names of many white doctors appeared, the lists invariably spotlighted the practices of well-known African American practitioners who represented a far greater proportion of their total numbers in the state than was the case for white doctors. The fact is hardly surprising. In 1969, Lloyd C. Elam, president of Meharry, estimated that 80 percent of the doctors who had trained at the school practiced in poverty areas.[22] NMA leaders warned that publication of such lists would make it hard to attract doctors to impoverished areas, and even the AMA joined in attacking the practice, not only because the lists were full of errors but because releasing the names of participants "serves only to badger a large segment of the profession and to establish guilt by innuendo."[23]

That possibility did not deter a white OBGYN specialist in Birmingham named Ronald E. Henderson, whose fiery accusations against the state's largest Medicaid providers found a sympathetic audience in the State Committee of Public Health on which he served and to which the director of the Medicaid program reported. Press accounts quoted him as denouncing the state attorney general's office for being insufficiently aggressive in rooting out Medicaid fraud and for not "looking into" its top earners, who, he asserted, did not deserve the money they were making. Offering no evidence to justify his demand, he insisted that the practices of the top ten Medicaid providers be "examined."[24]

The fact that the objects of Henderson's attacks included both midwives and numerous Black physicians for whom obstetrics formed a large part of their practices may have been more than coincidental. A sharecropper's son from the village of Prattville near Montgomery (his parents had been able to purchase 116 acres and a house there thanks to the New Deal's Farm Security Administration), Henderson trained at the University of Alabama. Young, cocksure, and gifted with a wealth of entrepreneurial talent, he soon became a young man on the go, first as head of obstetrics at Birmingham's St. Vincent's Hospital and then, in 1968, as founder and CEO of the Henderson and Walton Women's Center. Soon, his center had become the largest obstetrics practice in the southeast and by the early 1990s employed fifteen doctors in Birmingham and in seven other cities across the state, netting $12 million annually. "We were delivering 185 to 200 babies a month," he recalled in his autobiography.[25]

In February 1977, the legislature's Medicaid Study Committee subpoenaed five physicians whose earnings from the Medicaid program during the first quarter of the fiscal year ranked highest in the state. Although the stated purpose was to hear testimony on ways to improve Medicaid, the stigma attached to the subpoenas was obvious, even though the committee chair assured each recipient that "in no way are we suggesting that there has been any wrongdoing on your part."

The highest Medicaid earner was a white physician-lawyer in Bessemer who specialized in workmen's compensation and who had received $23,230 during the first quarter of the fiscal year. The next four were Black. In Huntsville, civil rights veteran Sonnie Wellington Hereford III was listed as having received $15,113. In Montgomery, Moses W. Jones, another civil rights veteran, earned $14,935. In Selma, Jesse J. Howard (who refused to appear) earned $13,441. In Mobile, pediatrician Judkin M. Robinson earned $11,640. Although they were not called to testify, three other Black doctors saw their names and earnings published as well, including Maynard V. Foster of Mobile, who was also active in civil rights ($10,341), William G. Reid of Tuskegee ($8,312), and Eyston A. Hunte of Prichard, a suburb of Mobile ($7,254).[26]

For these individuals, it was hard not to view the experience as anything other than an attempt to stigmatize Black health-care givers for whom Medicaid had introduced a modest degree of financial reward.

In 1978, the legislature created a Medicaid Fraud Control Unit, which was then placed in the office of the state attorney general. The following year, Charles A. Graddick Sr., newly elected to the post, began moving against those he suspected of Medicaid fraud, and the number of field investigations rose from twenty-seven in 1978 to sixty-seven in 1979. In the end, eleven Medicaid providers, several of them nursing home owners, were indicted, as was Dr. Hereford in Huntsville. His offense was that he billed for patients whom he had not personally attended. His explanation that the patients in question were being treated under a mutual arrangement with colleagues covering for him while he was out of town proved futile. Anxious over being tried in distant Montgomery and fearful of going to prison, he accepted a plea bargain in which he admitted guilt for two counts of Medicaid fraud while accepting probation and agreeing to pay back $150,000—twice the amount of the claims he had submitted.

Improper record keeping was among the leading ways that one could get into trouble with Medicaid investigators. The same was true for incorrect billing procedures. In 1970, a Yale law professor described Alabama's Medicaid reimbursement structure as one of the most complicated in the nation, in that one company paid for hospital and nursing home care, another for laboratory work and x-rays, and another for pharmaceuticals. For Black doctors, long accustomed to walk-in practices operating with a minimum of paperwork and often without sufficient staff to keep track of expanding numbers of Medicaid patients, errors were inevitable but were not necessarily proof of fraud.[27]

In early 1981, a new list, this one containing the names of doctors earning over $100,000 a year from Medicaid, appeared in newspapers across the state. Five of the eight physicians listed were Black. Of these, two had managed to build large practices in rural areas and appeared to be performing vital services in counties with few medical resources. One was a former Air Force medical officer named Robert X. Williams, an obstetrician in Macon County who served on the staff of Andrew Memorial Hospital and whose earnings were reported at $120,764. A Montgomery journalist described Williams's patients as being 90 percent "high risk, undernourished, needing special attention, sometimes extra hospitalization, and usually uninsured or underinsured. He might settle for $1 a month, but none were turned away."[28]

In the fall of 1987, after financial pressures forced Andrew Memorial to close its doors, Williams applied for privileges at the Bullock County Hospital in nearby Union Springs and promptly went to work in its long-closed obstetrical ward. According to the *Montgomery Advertiser*, the infant mortality rate in Bullock County soon dropped from 26.2 per thousand live births to 5.1. Because Williams was the only obstetrician in this part of the Black Belt, he literally worked himself to death, delivering between sixty and eighty babies a month. His son, a medical student at Meharry who sometimes assisted him, remembered how his father routinely put in sixteen to eighteen hours a day. In July of 1988, Dr. Williams collapsed in the operating room and died of a massive heart attack. Over one thousand mourners attended his funeral. "Our hospital changed with Dr. Williams," an administrator told the crowd. "It became a place of birth, of joy and happiness."[29]

The other rural Black doctor on the 1981 list was Earl Brown, who submitted 4,180 claims for a total of $121,468. While his practice was unusually large, Brown enjoyed a good reputation among both Black and white patients, as was evident in 1977 when officials of Lincoln, a majority-white community thirteen miles north of Talladega, recruited him for part-time duties in a new clinic being planned in an abandoned railroad depot and financed by a federal grant. Overburdened, Brown left after a year but was replaced by another Black doctor named William E. Davis, a Talladega native who had trained at Howard. Davis was at that time the only Black doctor in the county, and when money from the grant ran out, he transferred his private practice from Talladega to Lincoln and kept the clinic going. When Davis first arrived, the patient roster averaged ten a day; soon it was between thirty-five and forty. Davis also managed to transcend any racial divide as the clinic went from being 99 percent Black to 35 percent Black and 65 percent white.[30]

The other Black doctors on the 1981 list had built up large urban practices. In Montgomery, there was Moses Jones, who earned $107,764, and Robert McCorvey, who earned $126,367. McCorvey was an OBGYN specialist who had trained at Jefferson Medical College in Philadelphia; in the late 1970s, he gained notoriety among Alabama officials for suing the State Board of Corrections in federal court for its failure to provide adequate medical equipment at the Julia Tutwiler Prison for Women in nearby Wetumpka, where he served as part-time physician. He also complained that guards and matrons often contradicted his recommendations and that medical treatment for recaptured prisoners was often denied as a punishment.[31]

The highest Black earner on the list was an OBGYN specialist in Mobile named Winston H. Blake, who was reported to have earned $184,887 from Medicaid the previous year. A Howard graduate, Blake was a talented gynecologist who, in addition to overseeing a thriving practice in the Black suburb of Prichard, also served as a clinical instructor at the University of South Alabama College of Medicine. For Graddick, Blake was a tempting target, and just two months after the doctor's name appeared in the newspapers, he was charged with Medicaid fraud.

Dr. Blake's lawyer derided the accusation as political fodder for Graddick's coming campaign for governor. Indeed, for a crime that carried the possibility of prison, the charges seemed trivial—some urinalysis double-billings, which the lawyer described as simple clerical errors resulting from Medicaid paperwork, and a billing for a pap smear performed not in Blake's office but in a reference, or outside, laboratory. All other procedures, his lawyer said, were standard across the country. In the end, the jury agreed and found Blake innocent of all charges, but not before press coverage had damaged his reputation.[32]

In the meantime, the state legislature had created a new entity called the Medical Licensure Commission, which consolidated some of the profession's oversight powers into a group of seven physicians and one "consumer." Working hand-in-hand with the larger Board of Medical Examiners, the commission could subpoena witnesses, take depositions, and administer fines and reprimands. It also had authority to "issue, revoke, suspend and reinstate" any medical license in the state. Once in action, the commission worked to enforce professional standards and to terminate the practices of those deemed incompetent or guilty of gross negligence.

Black doctors sometimes found themselves facing sanctions, extending to the loss of their licenses. The charges typically involved unsafe prescribing practices, though in one case a Mobile practitioner was arrested for trying to trade drugs for sex to a female undercover officer. In Birmingham, a pediatrician lost his license for a felony conviction in federal court based on Medicaid fraud, while a Talladega internist was banned after he had allegedly engaged in unprofessional conduct resulting from "a mental or physical condition." A highly publicized case involved a Black doctor in Selma who attacked a colleague in the operating room of Good Samaritan Hospital. Jailed and permanently barred from the staff, the offender later opened a storefront clinic in Montgomery. Following complaints over the deaths of several babies he had delivered, medical authorities investigated eleven of his obstetrical cases and in 1988 revoked his license, accusing him of "an extraordinary lack of medical knowledge" for failing to provide infant warmers in his clinic and for sending mothers and babies home early, even when there had been respiratory or other problems.[33]

Incomplete figures from the automated database of the Alabama Board of Medical Examiners for the years 1960 to 2007 suggest that African Americans constituted around 11 percent of all physicians who were disciplined for assorted violations.[34] Findings published in 2000 by the Public Citizen's Health Research Group, which surveyed all doctors disciplined by the states or by the federal government over the previous nine years, showed that Alabama imposed a total of 366 disciplinary actions against physicians (some of these were multiple actions against the same person). Again, roughly 11 percent involved African Americans.[35]

Black doctors thus appear to have faced a disproportionate number of sanctions when compared with their white counterparts. It is not known whether their punishments were harsher than those imposed on white doctors—that is, whether white practitioners were more often able to avoid termination of their practices by instead receiving probation, fines, or letters of reprimand. In cases involving mental disorders, sexual misconduct, drug or alcohol addiction, credit card fraud, or criminal convictions, medical authorities appear to have dealt with Black doctors and white doctors on an equal basis. Less easy to evaluate are accusations against African American practitioners regarding excessive prescribing of controlled drugs, which cost six of them their licenses between 1995 and 2000 alone. As to Medicaid, while one cannot discount the possibility that a few Black physicians may have been guilty of filing false or misleading claims, such was not the case for the vast majority who, long before the advent of federal health-care programs, had lived exemplary lives, often providing care for their poorest patients at little or no charge. Nevertheless, the visibility of those with large Medicaid and Medicare practices made them vulnerable to law enforcement efforts.[36]

THE AFFORDABLE CARE ACT OF 2010

The battle over Medicaid expansion under the Affordable Care Act (ACA) of 1910 represented a new chapter in Alabama's ongoing refusal to make health care accessible to its poorest citizens. The political stalemate that followed passage of the bill demonstrated the strength of the entrenched racial attitudes that Black doctors faced during the segregationist era as well as the widespread poverty that attended their practices. The same year in which the

ACA became law saw poverty levels in Alabama hovering at just under 19 percent; according to the Kaiser Family Foundation, the rate for white people was 13.2 percent; for Black people, 32.6 percent; and for Hispanic people, 30.2 percent. Such figures illustrated a grim fact of life for many citizens: Poverty was King in the Heart of Dixie.[37]

The goal of the ACA was to reduce the estimated 48.6 million Americans having no health insurance, of whom a large proportion were Black and Hispanic. Specifically, the law mandated the extension of Medicaid eligibility in each state to include not only children but every adult under age sixty-four whose income was less than 138 percent of the poverty level. The federal government would bear the costs of this expansion through 2016, after which its share would decrease to 90 percent and remain at that level thereafter. In addition, the ACA required creation of online health insurance exchanges in each state; for individuals who purchased one of the private plans in their state, and whose incomes fell significantly below the poverty level, federal subsidies or tax credits were to be available.

The ACA was set to be implemented in January 2014. By then, the US Supreme Court, while upholding the constitutionality of the law, had ruled against the Medicaid mandate, stipulating that it was a matter for the states to decide. At first, just twenty-six opted to expand their coverage. Alabama was not among them, despite the ACA's economic benefits. According to research carried out at UAB, expanding Medicaid would not only shrink the ranks of the uninsured but, with the stimulus of $12.5 billion in federal matching funds over the next six years, generate $20 billion in new economic activity and $950 million in new taxes.[38]

The state's Republican leadership remained unmoved. When the US Supreme Court upheld the ACA, Governor Robert J. Bentley, a board-certified physician and founder of Alabama Dermatology Associates, denounced the law as "an overreach by the federal government" and "the single worst piece of legislation to come out of Congress." MASA leaders joined in the chorus of denunciations, arguing that the ACA would endanger the quality and availability of medical care in the state. Bentley subsequently rejected Medicaid expansion in the state and washed his hands of any role in organizing its health-care exchanges, which he left to the federal government.

Within MASA, opposition to the ACA hardly wavered during the ten years that followed, its leaders remaining focused not on the state's unfavorable national rankings in health-care availability but on professional concerns like tort reform and reducing regulatory burdens on doctors. Nor was MASA shy about using its financial clout to support political candidates who would help it maintain its rights and privileges. According to the nonprofit National Institute on Money in State Politics, MASA over a period of twenty-three years employed eleven different lobbyists and spent a total of $6,008,769 in contributions to 379 people who filed for political office. Included was one of $417,382 to the gubernatorial campaign of Robert J. Bentley in 2010.[39]

As time passed, MASA's longstanding opposition to federal involvement in medical practice began to weaken, a reflection no doubt of demographic changes in Alabama's medical corps as a whole. By 2021, African Americans and other physicians of color accounted for 22.8 percent of the total: specifically, there were 783 African Americans (7.1 percent); 1,191 who identified as Asian (10.8 percent), 338 as Hispanic (3.1 percent), 59 as American Indian or Alaskan Native (0.5 percent); and 145 of other races or ethnicities (1.3 percent).

Moreover, women now numbered 3,212, or 29 percent of all physicians, up from 24.6 percent in 2012.[40] They included individuals of extraordinary talent who spent much of their lives providing health care for poor people. Among them was Sandral Hullett, who practiced family medicine at the county hospital of tiny Eutaw and in 2001 became CEO of Birmingham's Cooper Green Mercy Hospital, the first Black woman in the state to serve as a hospital CEO. There was also UAB-trained Jacqueline Lewis, who joined Birmingham's Princeton Baptist Medical Center in 1992 and is regarded as the first Black female general surgeon in the state.

A breakthrough in the history of MASA occurred in 2002 with the election of Regina M. Benjamin to its presidency, the first African American to hold the position and the first to preside over a state medical society in the United States. A native of Mobile, Benjamin started her training at the Morehouse School of Medicine and continued at UAB and then the Medical Center of Central Georgia before she completed a residency in family medicine. Among her most impressive achievements was her service as a country doctor at the clinic she founded in Bayou La Batre, a small fishing and ship-building village located in Mobile County near the Gulf of Mexico.

Over time, Benjamin became involved in both MASA and the AMA as a means, she said later, to improve the care of her patients. In recognition of her service, the Kaiser Family Foundation awarded her its Nelson Mandela Award for Health and Human Rights in 2007. A year later, she received a MacArthur Fellowship, using the $500,000 that came with it to help rebuild her clinic, which had suffered from repeated hurricane damage. Then, in

2009, President Barack Obama nominated Benjamin to be the 18th US Surgeon General, a position she held for four years.

Dr. Benjamin was not the last person of color to serve as MASA president. In 2018, Jefferson Underwood III was elected to the position, his father having been among the first Black doctors to gain admittance to the Montgomery County Medical Society. In 2021, it was the turn of Huntsville neurologist Aruna T. Arora, the first Asian American in the post. She wasted little time in urging citizens to get vaccinated for COVID-19 and in trying to convince state legislators to expand Medicaid.

By now, women, African Americans, and Asian Americans were increasingly visible in the ranks of MASA's major committees, a fact that no doubt contributed to the organization's decision in 2020 to abandon its opposition to Medicaid expansion. In joining the Cover Alabama Coalition, which was made up of one hundred civic, religious, and health-care groups working toward this goal, MASA aligned itself with several activist groups long committed to racial equality, among them the Alabama NAACP, the Alabama Poor People's Campaign, and the Southern Poverty Law Center. It was a development that would have pleased the African Americans who braved the practice of medicine during the Jim Crow era, but one that few could have imagined.

Our study of Alabama's Black doctors during the century and a half following the end of Reconstruction presents compelling evidence of the discriminatory treatment accorded to African Americans trying to develop medical practices. Theirs is a story of both struggle and achievement, often at great personal costs, and it provides an essential context for understanding why reformers of the 1960s and 1970s sought to use affirmative action as a way to address the wrongs inflicted on Black physicians by Alabama's medical and political elites.

The attacks on affirmative action accompanying the conservative political resurgence of the modern era have also attempted to devalue diversity as a social benefit. Yet medical researchers have long stressed the importance of understanding racial and cultural differences in medical practice, which can strengthen a physician's empathy toward patients from all walks of life. Two educational researchers who have explored the effects on medical recruitment among students of color in states that have banned affirmative action stress the loss in practical terms as well, in that personal interactions with peoples of different colors and ethnicities serve to enhance "the learning and cross-cultural competencies of all doctors." The point is critical, given the nation's changing demographics and the fact that by the mid-twenty-first century minority populations will have exceeded 50 percent.[41]

Related to this is the well-documented tendency of both Black and Hispanic physicians to practice in medically underserved areas at a greater rate than other ethnic groups, as well as the preference of patients belonging to these minorities to be treated by physicians with whom they share a common racial or ethnic heritage.[42] As we have seen, during the Jim Crow era, some middle-class African Americans preferred white doctors, but that pattern changed as Black doctors gained access to hospitals with modern laboratories and lifesaving equipment and as they began to develop specialties.

As a result, African Americans of all social classes began to seek out Black physicians. "As a general rule," Duke psychiatrist Damon Tweedy noted in 2015, "Black patients are more likely to feel comfortable with Black doctors. Studies have shown that they are more likely to seek them out for treatment, and to report higher satisfaction with their care." Tweedy based his observations on his work in free clinics serving impoverished Black communities, where those who came seeking help specifically asked to see a Black doctor. The most convincing evidence, Tweedy added, was in the field of mental health, where Black patients being treated by white doctors were only half as likely as their white patients to receive care for behavioral disorders of comparable severity.[43]

Along with the historical analysis presented here, our oral accounts illustrate the human costs of segregation. That point was also among the findings of a group of historians and medical ethicists commissioned by the AMA in 2005 to trace the history of African Americans and the medical profession. Their report stressed that the racially exclusionist policies followed by the AMA and its constituent societies continue to have repercussions, as reflected in persistent health disparities affecting African Americans. Moreover, despite the tendency of many children of medical practitioners to follow in their parents' footsteps, the denial of equal opportunities to Black doctors may well have dissuaded many young African Americans from entering the profession. In the words of the report: "Many physicians follow relatives into medicine. As a result of this legacy of exclusion, generations of African Americans were not merely denied opportunities for basic and specialty training in medicine; they were largely denied familial examples as well."[44]

The history of Alabama's Black physicians, largely forgotten by younger generations, shows an enduring spirit of courage. The ability of our doctors to sustain an early love of biology or chemistry in the Black schools of their youth offers inspiration to young people of all races and backgrounds, a much-needed counterpoint to the drumbeat of popular culture and its sports and entertainment heroes. The tragedy of unequal access to health care and the continued underrepresentation of African Americans in the medical profession make further study of the history of Black health-care givers of great significance. Building on foundations laid over the past few decades with studies ranging from midwifery to the Black hospital movement to Black women's health activism, this story must be integrated into a broader history of local elites whose political values and economic interests have often proved injurious to the health and well-being of America's minorities and the poor.

Appendix

Select List of Black Hospitals in Alabama, 1890–1960

BIRMINGHAM

George C. Hall Hospital (1912), Dr. Ulysses G. Mason
Tuggle Institute Hospital (1920), Dr. Pierce S. Moten
Children's Home Hospital (1922), Smithfield, Children's Home Hospital Association
Southside Clinic (1932), Dr. Pierce S. Moten
Slossfield Health Center (1939), federal government
Holy Family Hospital (1943, expanded 1954), Ensley, Sisters Of Charity

DECATUR

Cottage Home Infirmary (1900), Dr. Willis E. Sterrs

MOBILE

Harris Infirmary (1910), Dr. Thomas N. Harris
Martin de Porres Hospital (1950), Sisters of Mercy

MONTGOMERY

Hale Infirmary (1890), Dr. Cornelius Nathaniel Dorsette
Northcross Sanatorium (1910), Doctors David C. Northcross Sr. and Daisy Hill Northcross
Fraternal Hospital Nursing School (1919), Frances Richardson
St. Jude Hospital (1951), Vincentian Sisters of Charity

SELMA

Burwell Infirmary (1907), Dr. Lincoln L. Burwell
Good Samaritan Hospital (1922, expanded 1947 and 1957), Sisters of St. Joseph

TALLADEGA

E. A. Goodnow Hospital (1910), Talladega College, Dr. William H. Brummit

TUSKEGEE

Tuskegee Institute Hospital (1892)
John A. Andrew Memorial Hospital (1913), Tuskegee Institute
Tuskegee Veterans Administration Hospital (1923)

Notes

PREFACE

1. Didier Fassin, *L'Espace politique de la santé: Essai de généalogie* (Paris: Presses Universitaires de France, 1996), 43. See also Jacques Léonard, "Les Médecins de l'ouest au XIXème siècle. Thèse presentée devant l'université de Paris le 10 janvier 1976," 3 vols. Lille: Atelier reproduction des theses, université de Lille III. Diffusion, Paris: Honoré Champion 1978; *La France médicale au XIXé siècle* (Paris: Editions Gallimard/Julliard, 1978); *La Médecine entre les saviors et les pouvoirs* (Mayenne: L'Imprimerie Floch, 1981); and Edward H. Beardsley, *A History of Neglect: Health Care for Blacks and Mill Workers in the Twentieth-Century South* (Knoxville: The University of Tennessee Press). See also W. M. Byrd and Linda A. Clayton, "Race, Medicine, and Health Care in the United States: A Historical Survey," *JAMA* 93 (March 2001): 11S-54s.

2. W. E. B. Dubois, *The Health and Physique of the Negro American* (Atlanta, GA: The Atlanta University Press, 1906), 73–90, 110; and Edwin T. Witt, *Witt's End* (Victorville, CA: E&C Publishers, 1997), 234–36.

3. W. Michael Byrd and Linda A. Clayton, *An American Health Dilemma: Race, Medicine, and Health Care in the United States, 1900–2000* (New York and London: Routledge, 2002), 158; and Mitchell F. Rice and Woodrow Jones Jr., "Black Health Inequities and the American Health Care System," *Health Policy and Education* 3 (1982): 195–214.

CHAPTER ONE

1. "Address by Dr. U. G. Mason, Birmingham, Alabama," *JNMA* 5 (July–September 1913): 151–53.

2. John A. Kenney, "Our Hospital: A Factor in the Prevention and Treatment of Disease," *JNMA* 5 (April–June 1913): 77–81. See also Eugene H. Dibble Jr., "The John A. Andrew Memorial Hospital," *JNMA* 22 (July–September 1930): 137–39; and Eugene H. Dibble Jr., Louis A. Rabb, and Ruth B. Ballard, "John A. Andrew Memorial Hospital," *JNMA* 53 (March 1961): 103–18.

3. John A, Kenney, "Isn't It Strange?" *JNMA* 3 (April–June 1931): 88–89.

4. Susan M. Reverby, *Examining Tuskegee: The Infamous Syphilis Study and Its Legacy* (Chapel Hill: University of North Carolina Press, 2009), 204.

5. Robert J. Norrell, *Up from History: The Life of Booker T. Washington* (Cambridge, MS: The Belknap Press of Harvard University Press, 2009), 121–35.

6. Norrell, *Up from History*, 1–16.

7. Louis R. Harlan, *The Booker T. Washington Papers Volume 2: 1860–89* (Urbana and Chicago: University of Illinois Press, 1972), 191–95.

8. *Howard University Record. Booker T. Washington* (Washington, DC: Howard University Press, 1909), 13–16. For Washington's comments on medicine and health, see Harlan and Raymond W. Smock, *The Booker T. Washington Papers Volume 10: 1909–11* (1981), 298–301; Harlan and Smock, *Volume 11, 1911–12* (1981), 407–10; and Harlan and Smock, vol. 13, *1914–15* (1984), pp. 268–69.

9. See the biographical sketch in W. Montague Cobb, "Cornelius Nathaniel Dorsette, M. D., 1852–1897," *JNMA* 52 (November 1960): 456–59.

10. Harlan, *The Booker T. Washington Papers Volume 4: 1895–98* (1975), 219–20.

11. Medical Association of the State of Alabama, *Transactions* (Montgomery, AL: Barrett & Brown, 1880), 97.

12. Harlan, *The Booker T. Washington Papers*, 2:501.

13. Harlan, *The Booker T. Washington Papers Volume 3: 1889–95* (1974), 186.

14. Harlan, *The Booker T. Washington Papers*, 3:164–67.

15. Alabama Department of Archives and History, State Board of Medical Examiners, application for certificate of qualification to practice medicine, 1879–1912, GR-BME-1, SG006464.

16. For a listing of early Black medical colleges, see Todd L. Savitt, "Four African-American Proprietary Medical Colleges: 1888–1923," *Journal of the History of Medicine* 55 (July 2000): 203–53.

17. Houston Brummit, *Talladega Days. Race, Rural Life, and Memories of a Forgotten Legend and KKK Survivor* (Bloomington, IN: iUniverse, 2011), 67.

18. Alabama Department of Archives and History, State Board of Medical Examiners, application for certificate of qualification to practice medicine, 1879–1912, GR-BME-1, SG006457.

19. Brummit, *Talladega Days*, 81.

20. Of eleven Black candidates who chanced the state boards between 1878 and 1891—five from Meharry and six from Howard—only four passed. See Medical Association of the State of Alabama, *Transactions* (Montgomery, AL: Brown Printing Company, 1892), 45–46.

21. See Grace Hooten Gates, "The Black Community," in *The Model City of the New South: Anniston, Alabama, 1872–1900* (Tuscaloosa: University of Alabama Press, 1996), 174–88. See also Ellen Griffith Spears, *Baptized in PCBs: Race, Pollution, and Justice in an All-American City* (Chapel Hill: University of North Carolina Press, 2014), 29–30.

22. *The Anniston Star*, July 22, 1993.

23. Alabama Department of Archives and History, Alabama State Board of Medical

Examiners, application for certificate of qualification to practice medicine, 1879–1912, GR-BME-1, SG006477.

24. *Proceedings of the National Negro Business League. Its First Meeting, Held in Boston, Massachusetts, August 23 and 24, 1900* (Boston, MA: J. R. Hamm, 1901), 66–71.

25. A. E. West, "Surgery in the Rural Districts: Some Helpful Hints," *JNMA* 10 (January–March 1918): 25–31. See also Loring B. Palmer, "Major Surgery in the Home," *JNMA* 10 (April–June 1918): 66–67.

26. Alabama Department of Archives and History, State Board of Medical Examiners, application for certificate of qualification to practice medicine, 1879–1912, GR-BME-1, SG006456.

27. C. M. Stevans, "The Race Problem in America: What the Negro Is Doing about It," *Our Day: A Record and Review of Current Thought and Action* 20 (September 1901): 225.

28. *The Pittsburgh Courier*, April 8, 1910. See also "Report of Committee on Medical Education on Colored Hospitals," *JNMA* 2 (October–December 1910): 283–90.

29. Brummit, *Talladega Days*, 61–64, 77.

30. Kenney, "The Hospital Ideal Essentially Altruistic," *JNMA* 4 (July–September 1912): 193–99, and "Report of Committee on Education on Colored Hospitals."

31. Harlan, *The Booker T. Washington Papers*, 13:303–4.

32. Alabama Department of Archives and History, State Board of Medical Examiners, GR-BME-1, SG6464. See also "The Profession and Conservation of Negro Health: President's Annual Address," *JNMA* 6 (October–December 1914): 215–21.

33. See Roscoe C. Brown, "The National Negro Health Week Movement," *The Journal of Negro Education* 6 (July 1937): 553–64.

34. John A. Kenney, "The Late Booker T. Washington: Friend of the Negro Physician," *JNMA* 38 (November 1946): 225–26.

35. "Were Most Successful Operations," *JNMA* 5 (January–March 1913): 53.

36. "Minutes of the John A. Andrew Clinical Society," *JNMA* 10 (April–June 1918): 89–96.

37. A detailed account of the meeting may be found under the "Society and Personal" section of the *JNMA* 13 (April–June 1921): 134–38. See also John A. Kenney, "Twenty-two Years of Public Health Work," *JNMA* 16 (April–June 1924): 131–34.

38. Kenney, "Isn't It Strange?" and "The Negro's Contribution to Surgery," *JNMA 33* (September 1941): 203–14.

39. David H. C. Scott, "Annual Address," *JNMA* 2 (April–June 1910): 96–101.

40. Glen Feldman, *Politics, Society, and the Klan in Alabama, 1915–1949* (Tuscaloosa: The University of Alabama Press, 1999), 7, 92–115, 133, 280.

41. See Vanessa Northington Gamble, *Making a Place for Ourselves: The Black Hospital Movement 1920–1945* (New York and Oxford: Oxford University Press, 1995), 70–104. For further information on the TVAH, see Eugene H. Dibble Jr., "Care and Treatment of Negro Veterans at Tuskegee," *JNMA* 35 (September 1943): 166–70; Clifton

O. Dummett and Eugene H. Dibble [Jr.], "Historical Notes on the Tuskegee Veterans Hospital," *JNMA* 54 (March 1962): 133–38; and Howard W. Kenney and Julian W. Giles, "Tuskegee Veterans Administration Hospital—Present and Future," *JNMA* 54 (March 1962): 139–45.

42. See appeals to NMA members for the names of qualified Black physicians in *JNMA 15* (July–September 1923): 203–4 and *JNMA* 16: (July-September 1924): 203.

43. Gamble, *Making a Place for Ourselves*, 90.

44. Gamble, *Making a Place for Ourselves*, 100. For a description of the early TVAH surgeons, see *A Century of Black Surgeons: The USA Experience*, eds. Claude H. Organ Jr. and Margaret M. Kosiba, vol. 1 (Norman, OK: Transcript Press, 1987), 337–53.

45. Ward, *Black Physicians in the Jim Crow South*, 275–77. See also "Dr. Jackson and the Tula Riots," *JNMA* 13 (July–September 1921): 202–3; and J. William Harris, "Etiquette, Lynching, and Racial Boundaries in Southern History," *American Historical Review* 100 (April 1995): 387–410.

46. See the recollections of Dr. Darden's nieces, Norma Jean and Carole Darden, in *Spoonbread and Strawberry Wine* (New York: Main Street Books, 1994), 40–41, 55, 150–51.

47. Dr. David C. Northcross Jr., interview by Jack D. Ellis from Atlanta, Georgia, January 4, 2000; and Ophelia Burnett Northcross, interview by Jack D. Ellis from Detroit, Michigan, January 5, 2000.

48. Marguerite W. Franklin, interview by Jack D. Ellis, Mobile, Alabama, October 21, 1998. See also Theodore Kornweibel, *Investigate Everything : Federal Efforts to Compel Black Loyalty during World War I* (Bloomington: Indiana University Press, 2002), 233.

49. Franklin, interview. See also Roy Hoffman's essay, "Dr. James Franklin: Healing Us Still," *Mobile Register*, October 13, 1996.

50. Details on Dr. Thomas's case are taken from his appeal before the Supreme Court of Alabama of May 18, 1908. See *The Southern Reporter, Containing All the Decisions of the Supreme Courts of Alabama, Louisiana, Florida, Mississippi, August 8, 1908–February 6, 1909*, vol. 47 (St. Paul, MN: West Publishing Company, 1909), 257–60.

51. Houston Brummit, *Talladega Days*, 71–74.

52. *The Chicago Defender*, May 10, 1924. See also *The New York Age*, May 17, 1924; and Brummit, *Talladega Days*, 129–42.

53. Savitt, "Entering a White Profession." See also Daniel M. Johnson and Rex R. Campbell, *Black Migration in America: A Social Demographic History* (Durham, NC: Duke University Press, 1981), 74–77, 96, 116.

54. Seale Harris, "The Future of the Negro from the Standpoint of the Southern Physician," *The Alabama Medical Journal* 14 (January 1902): 57–68.

55. Hale Tanner Dillon, "The Lafayette Dispensary in Connection with the Tuskegee Normal and Industrial Institute" (May 1894), The Legacy Center, Drexel University College of Medicine Archives and Special Collections, accessed September 25, 2023.

56. Robert S. Johnson, *Shadow of the Plantation* (University of Chicago Press, 1934), pp. 103–4, 148, 192–202. See also Reverby, *Examining Tuskegee*, 29–30.

57. Alabama Department of Archives and History, State Board of Medical Examiners, application for certificate of qualification to practice medicine, 1879-1912, GR-BME-1, SG006687.

58. William H. Frazier, MD, "Negro School Children in Tuskegee: Their Health and Their Environment," *Opportunity: A Journal of Negro Life* 13–14 (December 1935): 360–63.

59. Reverby, *Examining Tuskegee*, 36.

60. For an overview of the study, see Reverby, *Examining Tuskegee*, 1–10.

61. Fred Gray, *The Tuskegee Syphilis Study: The Real Story and Beyond* (Montgomery, AL: NewSouth Books, 1998), 1.

62. Calvin R. Dowe, interview by Jack D. Ellis, Tuskegee, Alabama, October 15, 1998.

63. John Franklin Hume, interview by Jack D. Ellis, Tuskegee, Alabama, October 14, 1998.

64. Calvin R. Johns Jr., interview by Jack D. Ellis, Montgomery, Alabama, October 27, 1998.

65. On Dibble's role, see Reverby, *Examining Tuskegee*, 152–66. See also James H. Jones, *Bad Blood: The Tuskegee Syphilis Experiment* (New York: The Free Press, 1993), 138, 145–50.

66. Susan M. Reverby, ed., *Tuskegee's Truths: Rethinking the Tuskegee Syphilis Study* (Chapel Hill: University of North Carolina Press, 2000), 57, 90–93, 159–60.

67. Gray, *The Tuskegee Syphilis Study*, 24, 62–64.

68. Mary Kaplan, *The Tuskegee Veterans Hospital and Its Black Physicians: The Early Years* (Jefferson, NC: McFarland & Company, 2016), 104.

69. Swope, interview.

70. Jones, *Bad Blood*, 81, 107.

71. Susan L. Smith, "Neither Victim Nor Villain: Eunice Rivers, the Tuskegee Syphilis Experiment, and Public Health Work," *Journal of Women's History* (Spring 1996): 95–113.

72. John A. Kenney, "The John A. Andrew Clinical Society: Adieu," *JNMA* 36 (March 1944): 60–61.

73. B. B. Wolcott, "Alabama Heals Her Crippled Children," *The Crisis*, February 1940.

74. Hume, interview.

75. John W. Chenault, "The Crippled Child," *JNMA* 28 (August 1936): 124–26. See also Edith Powell (Chappell) and John F. Hume, *A Black Oasis: Tuskegee Institute's Fight Against Infantile Paralysis* (March of Dimes Birth Defects Foundation, 1987), 29. Naomi Rogers presents an excellent scholarly overview in "Race and the Politics of Polio: Warm Springs, Tuskegee, and the March of Dimes," *American Journal of Public Health* 97 (May 2007): 784–95.

76. Eugene H. Dibble Jr., Louis A. Rabb, and Ruth B. Ballard, "John A. Andrew Memorial Hospital," *JNMA 53* (March 1961): 195; and Rogers, "Race and the Politics of Polio."

77. Hume, interview.

78. Powell and Hume, *A Black Oasis*, 51–52. See also *The Infantile Paralysis Fight at Tuskegee* (White Plains, NY: National Foundation for Infantile Paralysis, 1945), 24.

79. Hume, interview.

80. Howard W. Kenney and Julian W. Giles, "Tuskegee Veterans Administration Hospital—Present and Future," *JNMA* 54 (March 1962): 39–45.

81. See Kenney and Giles, "Tuskegee Veterans Administration Hospital," 133–173.

82. Henry W. Foster Jr. and Alice Greenwood, *Make a Difference* (New York: Scriber, 1997), 56–57, 83–85.

83. Foster, *Make a Difference*, 84–103.

84. Fred Gray, *Bus Ride to Justice: Changing the System by the System, the Life and Works of Fred Gray* (Montgomery, AL: Black Belt Press, 1995), 248–49.

85. Richard A. Serrano, "Tuskegee Still Holds Dr. Foster in Its Heart," *Los Angeles Times*, February 19, 1995.

86. *The Anniston Star*, June 19 and July 20, 1971.

87. Foster, *Make A Difference*, 163–64.

CHAPTER TWO

1. See Edward Magdol, *A Right to the Land: Essays on the Freedmen's Community* (Westport, CT: Greenwood Press, 1977), 211–13, 216–17; and Loren Schweninger, "A Vanishing Breed: Black Farm Owners in the South, 1651–1982," *Agricultural History* 63 (Summer 1989): 41–60.

2. Charles E. McGruder, interview by Jack D. Ellis, Nashville, Tennessee, October 1, 1998.

3. See Clifton Orrin Dummett, *The Growth and Development of the Negro in Dentistry in the United States* (Chicago, IL: The Stanek Press, 1952), 16, 19, 21–27, 77–82.

4. Alexander Lee Brewer, interview by Jack D. Ellis, Birmingham, Alabama, July 21, 1999.

5. McGruder, interview.

6. See the reprint of Mann's book in *Studies in American Negro Life: Negro Education in Alabama: A Study in Cotton and Steel*, ed. August Meier (New York: Atheneum, 1969), 256–58. See also James T. Patterson, *Brown v. Board of Education: A Civil Rights Milestone and Its Troubled Legacy* (Oxford and New York: Oxford University Press, 2001), xvii, 9; and table 6.6 in *The Education of Blacks in the South*, James D. Anderson (Chapel Hill and London: The University of North Carolina Press, 1988), 237.

7. Michael Fultz, "Teacher Training and African American Education in the South," *The Journal of Negro Education* 64 (Spring 1995): 196–210.

8. James T. Montgomery, interview by Jack D. Ellis, Birmingham, Alabama, October 28, 1998.

9. Montgomery, interview.

10. Tyree James Barefield-Pendleton, interview by Jack D. Ellis, Birmingham, Alabama, July 20, 1999.

11. The white owner of the land where the family sharecropped and who maintained a store where tenants were typically in debt.

12. Hagalyn Seay Wilson, interview by Jack D. Ellis, Montgomery, Alabama, October 27, 1998.

13. McGruder, interview.

14. McGruder, interview.

15. Hereford and Ellis, *Beside the Troubled Waters*, 23.

16. Montgomery, interview.

17. Jefferson Underwood Jr., interview by Jack D. Ellis, Montgomery, Alabama, October 26, 1998. See also Sharon G. Pierson, "New Perspectives on Progressive Education: HBCU Lab High Schools during Jim Crown," in *Contemporary Perspectives on African American Educational History*, eds. Dionne Danns, Michelle A. Purdy, and Christopher M. Span (Charlotte, NC: Information Age Publishing, Inc., 2015), 87–116.

18. McGruder, interview.

19. Hereford and Ellis, *Beside the Troubled Waters*, 24–25.

20. Flexner, *Medical Education in the United States and Canada*, 202, 307.

21. John J. Mullowney [president of Meharry], "Entrance Requirements to Meharry Medical College," *JNMA 16* (January–March 1924): 76–77; and Howard R. Epps, "The Howard University Medical Department in the Flexner Era: 1910–1929," *JNMA* 81 (August 1989): 885–911.

22. Carroll, interview.

23. Curry and Wilson, interviews.

24. Hereford and Ellis, *Beside the Troubled Waters*, 32.

25. Montgomery, interview.

26. Winston Jr., interview.

27. Montgomery, interview.

28. McGruder, interview.

29. Gunnar Myrdal, Richard Sterner, and Arnold Rose, *An American Dilemma: The Negro Problem and Modern Democracy* (New York and London: Harper & Brothers, 1944), 304–32.

30. Myrdal, *An American Dilemma*, 304–32; and J. Mills Thornton III, *Dividing Lines: Municipal Politics and the Struggle for Civil Rights in Montgomery, Birmingham, and Selma* (Tuscaloosa: University of Alabama Press, 2002), 178. See also the portrait of Arthur D. Shores by his daughters, Helen Shores Lee and Barbara S. Shores, in *The Gentle Giant of Dynamite Hill: The Untold Story of Arthur Shores and His Family's Fight for Civil Rights* (Grand Rapids, MI: Zondervan, 2012).

31. Montgomery, interview.

32. Hereford and Ellis, *Beside the Troubled Waters*, 22–23; and Thomas Edward Hereford, interview by Jack D. Ellis, Huntsville, Alabama, June 23, 2000.

33. Barefield-Pendleton, interview.

34. Hiram B. Moore, interviews by Jack D. Ellis, South Pittsburg, Tennessee, August 22 and September 26, 1997, and July 9, 1999.

35. Davis-Horton, *The Avenue*, 383; and *Atlanta Business Chronicle*, May 28, 2007.

36. Edwin T. Witt, *Witt's End* (Victorville, CA: E&C Publishers, 1997), 162–69.

37. John William Sherrer, interview by Jack D. Ellis, Anniston, Alabama, March 7, 2000.

38. Winston Jr., interview.

39. Wilson, interview.

40. Wilson, interview.

41. The names of women having received medical degrees from Meharry and Howard between 1872 and 1967 are found in *JNMA* 60 (March 1968): 152–55.

42. Dorothy L. Brown, interview by Jack D. Ellis, Nashville, Tennessee, September 19, 1997.

43. Underwood Jr., interview.

44. Brewer, interview.

45. Calhoun, interview.

46. See Margaret S. Klapper, "The Alabama Experience in Minority Recruitment," *JNMA* 65 (July 1973): 322–26.

47. Alex Carl Hansen, interview by Jack D. Ellis, Nashville, Tennessee, September 17, 1998.

48. Summerville, *Educating Black Doctors*, 86, 96–99.

49. Brewer, interview.

50. McGruder, interview.

51. J. L. B. Forrester, interview by Jack D. Ellis, Nashville, Tennessee, October 1, 1998. See also the analysis by Meharry registrar James R. Smother Jr. of students dropped for poor scholarship between 1938 and 1948, in *JNMA* 42 (January 1950): 46–47.

52. Curry, interview.

53. Barefield-Pendleton, interview.

54. Winston Jr., interview.

55. Barefield-Pendleton, interview.

56. Hereford and Ellis, *Beside the Troubled Waters*, 40.

57. Hereford and Ellis, *Beside the Troubled Waters*, 40; and J. L. B. Forrester, interview with Jack D. Ellis, Nashville, Tennessee, July 13, 2000.

58. McGruder, interview.

59. Summerville, *Educating Black Doctors*, 102, 121; and Hansen, interview.

60. Hansen, interview.

61. Barefield-Pendleton, interview.

62. See Thomas J. Ward Jr., *Out in the Rural: A Mississippi Health Center & Its War on Poverty* (New York: Oxford University Press, 2017), 76–77. See also *JNMA* 62 (July 1970): 306–09.

63. Charlotte Rose Walker, interview by Jack D. Ellis, Nashville, Tennessee, September 17, 1998.

64. Dowe, interview.

65. Calhoun, interview.

66. See Loretta J. Ross, "African-American Women and Abortion: A Neglected History," *Journal of Health Care for the Poor and Underserved* (Fall 1992): 274–284; Jessie M. Rodrique, "The Afro-American Community and the Birth Control Movement, 1918–1942" (PhD diss., University of Massachusetts Amherst, May 1991); and Leslie J. Reagan, *When Abortion Was a Crime: Women, Medicine, and the Law in the United States, 1867–1973* (Berkeley: University of California Press, 1997), 40–41, 48, 173.

67. For examples of highly publicized arrests for performing illegal abortions, see *The Tennessean,* October 4, 1939; April 1, 1948; March 5 and September 16, 1949; June 14, 1951; and July 9, 1953. See also Hugh Pearson, *Under the Knife: How a Wealthy Negro Surgeon Wielded Power in the Jim Crow South* (New York: The Free Press, 2000), 186; Hereford and Ellis, *Beside the Troubled Waters,* 44; and Reagan, *When Abortion Was a Crime,* 155.

68. Montgomery, interview.

69. Montgomery, interview.

70. See the letters of Pauline Dinkins to Dean Martha Tracy of June 22, 1919; Dean Tracy to Dinkins of June 30, 1919; and Dinkins to Dean Tracy of September 9, 1919, which are available online at Drexel Libraries E-Repository and Archives, Legacy Center Archives and Special Collections, College of Medicine.

71. Wilson, interview.

72. See "State Board Examinations for 1906," *The Journal of the American Medical Association* 48 (May 1907): 1781–87. See also H. F. Gamble, "Report on Medical Education," *JNMA* 2 (January–March 1910): 23–29.

73. See the tables in "Medical Licensure Statistics for 1946," in *The Journal of the American Medical Association* 134 (May 1946): 255–69.

74. Callis, "The Need and Training of Negro Physicians," 32–41.

75. See M. O. Bousfield, "Internships, Residencies and Postgraduate Training," *JNMA* 32 (January 1940): 224–30.

76. Numa P. G. Adams, "An Interpretation of the Significance of the Homer G. Phillips Hospital," *JNMA* 26 (February 1934): 13–17; and "Howard and Meharry Internship Appointments, 1972–73," *JNMA* 64 (September 1972): 459.

77. Dowe, interview.

78. Montgomery, interview.

79. Montgomery, interview.

80. Alma W. Foster, interview by Jack D. Ellis, Mobile, Alabama, October 23, 1998.

81. Curry, interview.

82. Wilson, interview.

83. The regions of practice described here are based on a modified version of those appearing in Bond's *Negro Education in Alabama*, 2–8.

84. See the description of Black neighborhoods in Glenn T. Eskew, *But for Birmingham: The National and Local Movements in the Civil Rights Movement* (Chapel Hill: University of North Carolina Press, 1997), 8–10, 63.

85. Theodore Rosengarten, *All God's Dangers: The Life of Nate Shaw* (New York: Vintage Books, 1974). Nate Shaw was the fictional name for Ted Cobb.

86. *The Birmingham News*, September 8, 1948.

87. See Byrd and Clayton, *An American Health Dilemma*, 231–32. For comparisons on specific diseases, see the tables in ibid., 366–77, and in David Baron Smith, *Health Care Divided: Race and Healing A Nation* (Ann Arbor: University of Michigan Press, 1999), 210–14. See also Winston Jr., interview.

CHAPTER THREE

1. Interview with Henry Hampton Brewer by Dr. William Bryant in *The Consortium: Concise History of Blacks in Medicine, 1983–1984*, 42–48, UAB Archives, MC54, Consortium.

2. Barefield-Pendleton, interview.

3. Underwood Jr., interview.

4. Ellen Tarry, *The Third Door: The Autobiography of an American Negro Woman* (New York: David McKay Company, 1955), 169–71.

5. *The Pittsburgh Courier*, June 1, 1953; and Taylor Branch, *Parting the Waters: America in the King Years 1953–63* (New York: Simon and Shuster, 1998), 15.

6. Underwood Jr., interview.

7. Winston, interview.

8. Wilson, interview.

9. Winston, interview.

10. See *The Birmingham News*, May 24, 1950, and *The Pittsburgh Courier*, August 12, 1950.

11. Curry, interview.

12. Montgomery, interview.

13. Montgomery, interview.

14. Moore, second interview (September 26, 1997).

15. Moore, first interview (August 22, 1997) and third interview (July 9, 1999).

16. Moore, second interview.

17. Hereford and Ellis, *Beside the Troubled Waters*, 70.

18. C. L. Marshall, "Racism and Health in Greene County, Alabama," *JNMA* 62 (March 1970): 109–14.

19. Barefield-Pendleton, interview.

20. Northcross, interview.

21. Swope, interview.

22. William A. Kates Jr., interview by Jack D. Ellis, Huntsville, Alabama, February 28, 2001.

23. Montgomery, interview.

24. Kates Jr., interview.

25. Barefield-Pendleton and Sherrer, interviews.

26. Underwood Jr., Hunte, and LeFlore, interviews.

27. Wilson, interview.

28. Rodgers Jr., interview.

29. Curry, interview.

30. Curry, interview.

31. Underwood Jr., interview.

32. Moore, first interview (August 22, 1997) and second interview (September 26, 1997).

33. Hereford and Ellis, *Beside the Troubled Waters*, 45; Barefield-Pendleton, interview.

34. Sherrer, interview.

35. Hereford and Ellis, *Beside the Troubled Waters*, 60.

36. Ibid., 124–25.

37. M. Alfred Haynes, "The Distribution of Black Physicians in the United States, 1967," *JNMA* 61 (November 1969): 470–73; and Calhoun, interview.

38. Winston Jr., interview; and Calvin R. Johns Jr., interview by Jack D. Ellis, Montgomery, Alabama, October 27, 1998.

39. Winston Jr., interview.

40. Jefferson Underwood III, interview by Jack D. Ellis, Montgomery, Alabama, October 26, 1998.

41. Underwood Jr., interview.

42. Sherrer, interview.

43. Montgomery, interview.

44. Barefield-Pendleton, interview.

45. Hereford and Ellis, *Beside the Troubled Waters*, 60–61.

46. Geneva Drake Whatley, interview by Jack D. Ellis, Huntsville, Alabama, July 26, 1999.

47. Underwood Jr., interview.

48. See the sketches of Wilson by Earl Thaxton in the *Montgomery Advertiser*, March 4, 1990, and by Teri Greene in ibid., August 31, 2001.

49. Wilson, interview.

50. Hereford and Ellis, *Beside the Troubled Waters*, 60–61.

51. Moore, second interview (September 26, 1997).

52. Montgomery, interview.

53. Moore, second interview.

54. Wilson, interview.

55. Hereford and Ellis, *Beside the Troubled Waters*, 66.

56. See John B. Houde, Beverly W. Boyd, and Robert L. Goldenberg, "Out of Hospital Deliveries in Alabama 1940–1980," *Journal of the Medical Association of the State of Alabama* 52 (August 1982): 20–25.

57. McGruder, interview.

58. Whatley, interview.

59. Whatley, interview.

60. Claudia M. Donalson, interview by Jack D. Ellis, Fayetteville, Tennessee, July 31, 1997.

61. Moore, third interview (July 9, 1999).

62. See Marla Schenck Melton, "Health Manpower and Negro Health: The Negro Physician," *Journal of Medical Education*, 43 (July 1968): 798–814.

63. See the estimate of gross incomes of NMA members by region in George E. Schwarz and Montague S. Lawrence, "Selected Characteristics of the National Medical Association: Preliminary Findings," *JNMA* 62 (January 1970): 1–7.

64. Hereford and Ellis, *Beside the Troubled Waters*, 56, 61–62.

65. Moore, second interview (September 26, 1997).

66. Barefield-Pendleton, interview.

67. Montgomery, interview.

68. Local Black doctors made up six of the bank's fifteen officers. See the *Mobile Register*, January 20, 1974.

69. Eyston A. Hunte, interview by Jack D. Ellis, Mobile, Alabama, October 21, 1998. See also the *Mobile Register*, June 20, 22 and July 20, 1984, and December 2, 1985.

70. Montgomery and Barefield-Pendleton, interviews.

71. Northcross, interview.

72. Carroll, interview.

73. Franklin, interview.

74. Barefield-Pendleton, interview.

75. Brewer, interview.

76. Curry, interview.

CHAPTER FOUR

1. See Douglas A. Blackmon, *Slavery by Another Name: The Re-Enslavement of Black Americans from the Civil War to World War II* (New York: Anchor Books, 2009).

2. Algernon Brashear Jackson, "Investigation of Negro Hospitals," *JAMA* 92 (April 1929): 1375–76; and Algeron Brashear Jackson, "Hospitals and Health," *JNMA* 22 (July–September 1930): 115–19. See also H. M. Green, "A Brief Study of the Hospital Situation Among Negroes," *JNMA* 22 (July–September 1930): 112–14.

3. See tables 1 and 2 in American Medical Association, Council on Medical Education, "Hospital Service in the United States for the Year 1920," *JAMA* 76 (16 April 1921): 1083–1103. For details on Alabama, see *The American Hospital Digest and Directory*, 3rd ed. (Chicago, IL: The Crain Publishing Company, 1930), 68–69.

4. See David Barton Smith, "The Politics of Racial Disparities: Desegregating the Hospitals in Jackson, Mississippi," *The Milbank Quarterly: A Multidisciplinary Journal of Population and Health Policy* 83 (June 2005): 247–69.

5. Leona Lyons, "Four Institutions Maintain 'Basement Hospitals' for Negroes here in Birmingham," *The Weekly Review*, July 18, 1941.

6. Albert W. Dent, "Hospital Services and Facilities Available to Negroes in the United States," *The Journal of Negro Education* 18 (Summer 1949): 326–32.

7. *The Enterprise Ledger*, February 6, 1958; and *The Semi-Weekly Advocate*, Greenville, Alabama, March 1, 1924.

8. *The Huntsville Times*, January 9, 1925.

9. Richard L. Lester Jr., interview by Jack D. Ellis, Huntsville, Alabama, January 20, 2000.

10. "Jefferson County's Study of Medical Care," *JMASA* 8 (January 1939): 259–63.

11. Lyons, "Four Institutions Maintain 'Basement Hospitals' for Negroes."

12. "Interview with Charles F. Zukoski Jr.," interview by Cliff Kuhn, September 9, 1984, in Working Lives Oral History Project, University of Alabama Libraries Special Collections.

13. For the census tracts of 1940 showing percentages of African American residents, see Charles E. Connerly, *"The Most Segregated City in America": City Planning and Civil Rights in Birmingham, 1920–1980* (Charlottesville: University of Virginia Press, 2013), 55, 104–8.

14. The brief autobiography by Moten, entitled "A Sketch of My Life and Work," is found in "Dr. Pierce S. Moten," *JNMA* 54 (July 1961): 432–35. For the work of Carrie Tuggle, see Lynne B. Feldman, *A Sense of Place: Birmingham's Black Middle-Class Community, 1890–1930* (Tuscaloosa: University of Alabama Press, 1999), 172–76.

15. "Dr. Pierce S. Moten."

16. Information on Moten's emergency station and the Southside Clinic that replaced it is found in the UAB Archives, MC53, folders 4.15 and 4.32. The collection was assembled by Mary Rhinelander McCarl, director of the Jefferson County Medical Society/University of Alabama at Birmingham Health Sciences Archives, between 1988 and 1990. Also included (folder 4.39) is McCarl's unpublished but highly informative article "A Hospital By and For Blacks: A Chapter in the Medical History of Birmingham, Alabama, 1930–1954," which won the Gottlieb Prize in the history of medicine from the Medical Library Association in 1991.

17. See Fallin Jr., *The African American Church in Birmingham, Alabama*, 98, 129. On Edmonds, see Sarah Woolfolk Wiggins, *From Civil War to Civil Rights, Alabama, 1860–1960: An Anthology from the Alabama Review* (Tuscaloosa: University of Alabama Press, 1987), 261, 268–70.

18. See the historical summary by Tim L. Pennycuff in the Slossfield Photograph Collection, 1933–1940, and a copy of an unsigned report from the Tutwiler Collection of the Birmingham Public Library entitled "Slossfield Health Center, 1940," UAB Archives, P08 and MC52 4.7.

19. Walter H. Maddux, "The Slossfield Health Center: An Example of Local Medical Service for Mothers and Children under Public Health Auspices," *American Journal*

of Public Health 31 (May 1941): 481–86; T. M. Boulware, Elizabeth LaForge, and R. C. Stewart, "A Negro Demonstration Center for Maternal and Newborn Care in Alabama," *Southern Medical Journal* 36 (December 1943): 748–91; and McCarl, "A Hospital By and For Blacks," UAB Archives, M53, 4.3.

20. Slossfield Health Center 1940, UAB Archives, MC53 4.7,1940; and Maddux, "The Slossfield Health Center," 481–90.

21. Maddux, "The Slossfield Health Center." In obstetrics, the names included Edward H. Ballard, Hampton Brewer, Nathaniel J. Broughton, Walter L. Brown, Lorenzo S. Demby, Samuel F. Harris, John E. Hutchinson, Cecil S. Giscombe, Herbert O. Matthews, Marion G. McCall, Aldus S. Mitchell, and Adolphus Wimbs Plump. Pediatrics included Ballard, Brewer, Brown, Broughton, William L. Drake, Giscombe, Matthews, and Plump.

22. Charles E. Connerly points out that in the 1940 census of the city's fifty-two tracts, fifteen were 75 percent or more Black, of which parts of seven were zoned for heavy industry. See *The Most Segregated City in America*, 53, and also table. 5.1 in "Black Population by Census Tract, 1940–1970," 152–53.

23. UAB Archives, MC53, 4.3

24. Maddux, "The Slossfield Health Center," 481–86.

25. Denison to Kracke, August 30, 1944, UAB Archives, MC53 4.34, 17.1.1.

26. Thomas M. Boulware, interview by Virginia Fisher, Birmingham, Alabama, June 30, 1987, UAB Archives, MC53, 4.15.

27. See James W. Stewart's account of his family and his own civil rights activities in Cynthia Levinson, *We've Got a Job: The 1963 Birmingham Children's March* (Atlanta, GA: Peachtree Publishers, 2012), 21–27.

28. Boulware, interview.

29. T. M. Boulware, Elizabeth LaForge, and R. C. Stewart, "A Negro Demonstration Center for Maternal and Newborn Care in Alabama," *Southern Medical Journal* 36 (December 1943): 748–91.

30. Alfred A. Walker et al., *A Report of the Jefferson County Board of Health Covering the Years 1943 and 1944* (August 1945), UAB Archives, MC53, 5.35.

31. Jennifer Nelson, "Healthcare Reconsidered: Forging Community Wellness among African Americans in the South," *Bulletin of the History of Medicine* 81 (Fall 2007): 594–624.

32. "Slossfield, MASA," UAB Archives, MC53, folder 4.3.

33. On Slossfield's closing, see Nelson, "Healthcare Reconsidered," and McCarl, "A Hospital By and For Blacks."

34. *The Birmingham News*, September 8, 1948.

35. "Slossfield, MASA," UAB Archives, MC53, folder 4.3.

36. For information on Kracke's career and the opening of the Medical College of Alabama, see Tennant S. McWilliams, *New Lights in the Valley: The Emergence of UAB* (Tuscaloosa: University of Alabama Press, 2007), 32–51.

37. See the NHA's "Receipts and Disbursements" report of September 1944 in UAB Archives, MC53, 4.34. See also Christopher MacGregor Scribner, *Renewing Birmingham: Federal Funding and the Promise of Change, 1929–1979* (Athens: University of Georgia Press, 2002), 40–43.

38. Denison to Kracke, August 30, 1944, UAB Archives, MC53, 4.34.

39. "Proposals on Policy of the Mineral District Medical Society as to Hospital Facilities Offered to Negroes in Birmingham," October 15, 1944, UAB Archives, MC53, 1.12.

40. Kracke to Birmingham and Jefferson County Negro Hospital Association, November 28, 1944, and Bishop Shaw to Kracke, 16 December 1944, UAB Archives, MC53, folder 4.34.

41. Denison to Kracke, December 5, 1945, UAB Archives, MC53, folder 1.13.

42. Kracke to Shaw, December 6, 1945, ibid.

43. Kracke to Shaw, December 6, 13, 1945, ibid.

44. "Interview with Charles F. Zukoski Jr."

45. See McWilliams, *New Lights in the Valley*, 62–68.

46. Toole to Kracke, March 20, 1945, UAB Archives, MC53, folder 1.14.

47. Kracke to Toole, March 23, 1946, UAB Archives, MC53, folder 1.14.

48. *The Weekly Review*, February 26, 1911; and Lyons, "Four Institutions Maintain 'Basement Hospitals' for Negroes."

49. See the description of Children's Home in "The Holy Family Hospital, Ensley, Alabama," *JNMA* 55 (January 1963): 86–88. See also *The Birmingham News*, March 20, 1943, and *The Weekly Review*, July 3, 1948.

50. Other doctors who frequented Children's Home were Henry Clay Bryant, Ransey G. Cole, Henry L. Dale, William L. Drake, Samuel F. Harris, Marion G. McCall, and Lionel F. Swan. See the description in "The Holy Family Hospital, Ensley, Alabama," *JNMA* 55 (January 1963): 86–88; and *The Consortium*, Hampton Brewer interview by William Bryant.

51. Brewer, interview.

52. Boulware, interview, 1987.

53. On details of the fund-raising campaigns, see Scribner, *Renewing Birmingham*, 43–49.

54. Kracke to Zukoski, July 31, 1948, and January 26, 1950, UAB Archives, MC53, folder 4.35.

55. "Interview with Charles F. Zukoski Jr."

56. Harrison to Zukoski, October 19, 1950, and to Louis D. Green, October 20, 1950, UAB Archives, MC53, folder 4.35.

57. *Detroit Free Press*, June 17, 1999.

58. *Birmingham News*, March 14, 23, 1951.

59. Emil C. Hess to Harrison, April 3, 1951, UAB Archives, MC53, folder 4.35. See also the *Birmingham News*, April 10, 1951.

60. Young Men's Business Club of Birmingham to Harrison, April 17, 1951, UAB Archives, MC53, folder 4.35.

61. Harrison to Emil C. Hess, April 6, 1951, UAB Archives, MC53, folder 4.35.

62. Harrison to Brewer Dixon, May 7, 1951, UAB Archives, MC53, folder 4.35.

63. *JMASA* 23 (July 1953): 27–28.

64. Roy R. Kracke and Arthur L. Bailey, "The Jefferson-Hillman Hospital," *JMASA* 20 (July 1950): 10–16.

65. Lyons, "Four Institutions Maintain 'Basement Hospitals' for Negroes Here in Birmingham."

66. Employees Hospital of the Tennessee Coal, Iron, and Railroad Company, a 319-bed hospital in Fairfield.

67. Brewer, interview.

68. Dodson M. Curry, tour of Black medical sites in Birmingham with Jack D. Ellis and Tim L. Pennycuff, February 8, 2000, Ellis Collection, UAB Archives; Herschell Lee Hamilton's comment is from the *Birmingham News*, April 17, 2000.

69. The others were Ferd D. Bradford Sr., Ferd D. Bradford Jr., Ransey G. Cole, William L. Drake, Cecil S. Giscombe, Louis D. Green, Samuel F. Harris, and Adolphus W. Plump. Younger physicians included Dodson M. Curry, Henry L. Dale, and Edwin T. Witt.

70. Dodson M. Curry, tour of Black Medical Sites in Birmingham with Jack D. Ellis and Tim L. Pennycuff, February 8, 2000.

71. Curry, interview; and Clay Norris Wells, *Please God, Don't Call Me to Preach* (New York: iUniverse, Inc., 2004), 78–79.

72. Curry, interview; and letter to Jack D. Ellis March 15, 2000, UAB Archives, Ellis Collection.

73. Montgomery, interview.

74. Sister Maria, "History of the Saint Martin de Porres Hospital, Mobile, Alabama," *JNMA* 56 (July 1964): 303–06.

75. LeFlore, interview.

76. Kendal I. Foster, interview by Jack D. Ellis, Mobile, Alabama, October 28, 1998.

77. Joy HP Harriman, *Health Care in Mobile: An Oral History of the 1940s* (CreateSpace Independent Publishing Platform, 2011), 98, 137, 192.

78. See Robert S. Wilkinson, "The Residency Training Program in General Surgery, Tuskegee Veterans Administration Hospital," ibid. 54 (March 1962): 149–151.

79. Harriman, *Health Care in Mobile*, 159; Franklin, interview; and *Mobile Register*, December 24, 1977.

80. See M. Joyce Barber, "A Tribute to James E. Caple," *JNMA* 86 (August 1994): 567.

81. Winston Jr., interview.

82. Underwood Jr., interview.

83. Underwood Jr., interview.

84. Barbra Mann Wall, "Catholic Sister Nurses in Selma, Alabama, 1940–1972,"

Advances in Nursing Science 32 (January–March 2009): 91–102; and Amy L. Koehlinger, *The New Nuns: Racial Justice and Religious Reform in the 1960s* (Cambridge: Harvard University Press, 2007), 1–4.

85. Completing Selma's small Black medical corps were the dentists J. H. Williams and a World War II veteran named Sullivan "Sully" Jackson. See Richie Jean Sherrod Jackson, *The House by the Side of the Road: The Selma Civil Rights Movement* (Tuscaloosa: The University of Alabama Press, 2011), 20–23.

86. Chestnut and Cass, *Black in Selma*, 140–41.

CHAPTER FIVE

1. Charles R. Drew, "Negro Physicians and the American Medical Association," *JNMA* 39 (September 1947): 222–24.

2. See Spencie Love, *One Blood: The Death and Resurrection of Charles R. Drew* (Chapel Hill and London: The University of North Carolina Press, 1996), especially 13–30, which describes the accident and its aftermath in detail.

3. Hyson Jr., "Doctors Five"; and the *St. Louis Globe-Democrat*, February 12, 1899.

4. *The Birmingham News*, December 2, 1899.

5. "The World War—What Does It Mean? How Does it Apply to the Afro-American?," *JNMA* 9 (October–December 1917): 195–97.

6. *The Montgomery Advertiser*, April 11, 1917, and October 11, 1918; and *The Birmingham News*, April 15, 1917.

7. *The Albany-Decatur Daily*, April 19, 1917. Depositions regarding events in Cuba appear in Herschel V. Cashin et al., *Under Fire with the Tenth U.S. Cavalry* (New York: Arno Press, 1969). See also Sheryll Cashin, *The Agitator's Daughter: A Memoir of Four Generations of One Extraordinary African-American Family* (New York: PublicAffairs, 2008), 47–63, 58–60.

8. *The Birmingham Reporter*, April 26, 1919.

9. *Our Mountain Home*, March 26, 1919; and Fisher and Buckley, *African American Doctors of World War I*, 122–24, 149–50. *Our Mountain Home* was a newspaper in Talladega, Alabama.

10. Rodgers Jr., interview.

11. Underwood Jr., interview.

12. Robert W. Gilliard, interviews by Jack D. Ellis, Mobile, Alabama, October 20, 21, 1998.

13. Kendal I. Foster, interview by Jack D. Ellis, Mobile, Alabama, October 21, 1998; and Alma W. Foster, interview.

14. Democrat Theodore G. Bilbo, twice governor of Mississippi and then US senator (1935–1947), a member of the Ku Klux Klan and militant defender of white supremacy. Barefield-Pendleton relates this anecdote and other details of his military experiences in J. Mack Lofton Jr., *Healing Hands: An Alabama Medical Mosaic* (Tuscaloosa and London: University of Alabama Press, 1995), 79–82.

15. Barefield-Pendleton, interview.

16. Barefield-Pendleton, interview.

17. Curry, interview.

18. Jacquelyn Dowd Hall, "The Long Civil Rights Movement and the Political Uses of the Past," *The Journal of American History* 91 (March 2005): 1233–63.

19. Rodgers Jr., interview. See also Kevern Verney, "'To Hope Till Hope Creates': The NAACP in Alabama, 1913–1945," in *Long Is the Way and Hard: One Hundred Years of the National Association for the Advancement of Colored People (NAACP)*, eds. Kevern Verney and Lee Sartain (Fayetteville: University of Arkansas Press), 105–120.

20. Barefield-Pendleton, interview.

21. John Dittmer, *Local People: The Struggle for Civil Rights in Mississippi* (Urbana and Chicago: University of Illinois Press, 1995), 46–47, 75–77; and *The Good Doctors: The Medical Committee for Human Rights and the Struggle for Social Justice in Heath Care* (New York: Bloomsbury Press, 2009), 31. See also Ward, *Black Physicians in the Jim Crow South*, 265–94.

22. Richard D. deShazo, ed., *The Racial Divide in American Medicine* (Jackson: University Press of Mississippi, 2018), 83–104.

23. Melanie S. Morrison, *Murder on Shades Mountain: The Legal Lynching of Willie Patterson and the Struggle for Justice in Jim Crow Birmingham* (Durham and London: Duke University Press, 2018), 134. See also Verney, "'To Hope Till Hope Creates': The NAACP in Alabama, 1913–1945"; and Wilson Fallin Jr., *The African American Church in Birmingham, Alabama, 1815–1963. A Shelter in the Storm* (New York and London: Garland Publishing, Inc., 1997), 126–27.

24. Feldman, *A Sense of Place*, 159; Verney and Sartain, *Long Is the Way and Hard*, 105–120; Robin D. G. Kelley, *Hammer and Hoe: Alabama Communists during the Great Depression* (Chapel Hill: University of North Carolina Press, 2015), 83–90, 124–25; and Morrison, *Murder on Shades Mountain*, 89–90.

25. Dan Carter, *Scottsboro: A Tragedy of the American South*, 200. Among other names on the list of thirty-one names were the Black physician Winston H. Sherard, the dentist J. W. Wood, and the pharmacist Arthur O. Sheffey, who had worked with the late Dr. Sterrs at Magnolia Drugstore. The list was discovered in 2007 by Morgan County archivist John Allison. See Deangelo McDaniel's report in *The Decatur Daily*, September 30, 2007. See also Cashin, *The Agitator's Daughter*, 74–77.

26. For further details throughout the South, see "Medical Society of Georgia Votes Restricted Membership for Negro Physicians" and "Fourteen Colored Physicians Join Florida Medical Association," *JNMA* 44 (July 1952): 316; "Georgia County Society Opens Doors Wide," *JNMA* 45 (January 1953): 75–76; "Charleston County (South Carolina) Medical Society Admits Negro Physicians," *JNMA* 45 (March 1953): 153–54; "Alabama Medical Association Votes to Admit Negroes," *JNMA* 45 (July 1953): 291; and "North Carolina Physicians Refuse Limited Membership," *JNMA* 49 (March 1957): 115.

27. *The Anniston Star*, June 11, 1950.

28. "Message of the President," *JMASA* 21 (May 1952): 340–43.

29. "On Membership Extension," *JMASA* 22 (June 1953): 347.

30. See "Dallas Hospitals Admit Five Negro Physicians to Staff," *JNMA* 46 (September 1954): 367, 370.

31. Whatley, interview.

32. Whatley, interview.

33. Hereford and Ellis, *Beside the Troubled Waters*, 59.

34. Joseph M. Dixon, who received his medical degree from the University of Virginia in 1935, was associate professor of ophthalmology at the Medical College of Alabama and vice-president of the Alabama Academy of Ophthalmology.

35. Brewer, interview.

36. Jones served as second vice president of the Montgomery Improvement Association and in February 1956 was arrested for his activities in support of the bus boycott.

37. Underwood Jr., interview.

38. Solomon S. Seay Jr., *Jim Crow and Me: Stories from My Life as a Civil Rights Lawyer* (Montgomery and Louisville: NewSouth Books, 2008), 82.

39. Underwood Jr., interview.

40. Sheryll Cashin, *The Agitator's Daughter*, 115–16.

41. The majority of those who signed bonds were Black businessmen. An undated mimeographed list of bond signers in Dr. Hereford's papers provides the names of eleven Black businessmen and one minister. Evelyn Howie, wife of the white pediatrician Virgil Howie, recalled that she herself signed over fifty bonds because the house was in her name. See Dr. Virgil Howie, Evelyn Howie, and Dr. William Goodson, joint interview by Jack D. Ellis, Huntsville, Alabama, September 24, 1999.

42. These events are treated in detail in Hereford and Ellis, *Beside the Troubled Waters*, 86–126.

43. *The Birmingham News*, April 17, 2000.

44. Eskew, *But for Birmingham*, 127.

45. *Birmingham Post-Herald*, April 23, 1963. The seventeen doctors who signed the statement were Tyree James Barefield-Pendleton, Depew E. Bradford, Ferdinand D. Bradford Sr., Ferdinand D. Bradford Jr., Alexander Lee Brewer, Henry Hampton Brewer, C. L. Burgess, William L. Drake, Herschell Lee Hamilton, Clarence R. Hixon, Samuel E. Harris, James T. Montgomery, Pierce S. Moten, Robert C. Stewart, Adolphus W. Plump, Joseph Wilburn Samuels Jr., and Herbert O. Matthews. The nine dentists were J. A. Boykin, Joel S. Boykin, W. J. Dowdell, Eugene L. Elliot Jr., R. M. Howard, Benjamin M. Jefferson, Aubrey Shakespeare, Ernest W. Taggart, and S. E. Welch.

46. Barefield-Pendleton, interview. Ruth Barefield-Pendleton was present for part of the interview and commented briefly on her activities in 1963.

47. Curry, interview.

48. Brewer, interview.

49. Montgomery, interview.

50. Wells, *Please God, Don't Call Me to Preach*, 117–18.

51. Underwood Jr., interview.

52. Wilson, interview.

53. See interview with Dr. William Dinkins conducted by Blackside, Inc. on September 13, 1979, for "Eyes on the Prize: America's Civil Rights Years (1954–1965)," Washington University Libraries, Film and Media Archive, Henry Hampton Collection.

54. Koehlinger, *The New Nuns*, 239.

55. Excerpts from Miller's diary are included in the sketch of Rev. Reeb's "A Good Man's Death" found in Jack Mendelsohn, *The Martyrs: Sixteen Who Gave Their Lives for Racial Justice* (New York: Harper and Row, 1966).

56. Dittmer, *The Good Doctors*, 93.

57. See "The National Medical Association's Contribution to the Selma-Montgomery March," *JNMA* 57 (May 1965): 243–45.

58. Gilliard, interviews.

59. *The Anniston Star*, January 8, 1967.

60. *Jet* magazine, May 19, 1966.

61. Smith, *Health Care Divided*, 155.

62. *The Southern Courier*, February 25–26, 1967.

63. *The Southern Courier*, December 31–January 1, 1967.

64. David Barton Smith provides an overview of these events in *Health Care Divided*, 154–59. See also Beatrix Hoffman, *Health Care for Some: Rights and Rationing in the United States since 1930* (Chicago, IL: University of Chicago Press, 2012), 126–27.

65. *Maynard V. Foster and LeBaron A. Foster v Mobile County Hospital Board et al.*, United States Court of Appeals, Fifth Circuit—June 24, 1968 (CA5 Ala) 398 F2d 227, 37 ALR3d 637; *American Law Reports, Annotated Third Series* (Bancroft-Whitney Company, 1971), 637–44.

66. An example was *Greisman v. Newcomb Hospital* in 1963, which involved a doctor of osteopathy, a branch of medicine not then recognized by the AMA. See *Maynard V. Foster and LeBaron A. Foster v Mobile County Hospital Board et al.*, 645–703.

67. *The Southern Courier*, August 13, 1965.

68. *The Anniston Star*, December 31, 1950, and January 9, 1951.

69. *The Anniston Star*, March 20 and June 22, 1965.

70. *The Southern Courier*, December 11–12, 1965.

71. *Report of U.S. Commission on Civil Rights*, February 1966, 5–6, 11–12, 13.

72. Montgomery, interview.

73. Brewer, interview.

CHAPTER SIX

1. Association of American Medical Colleges (AAMC), *Diversity in the Physician Workforce: Facts & Figures* 2010, tables 13 and 14a, 81–82. Unless otherwise noted, the statistical information cited in the final chapter is taken from maps and tables provided in periodic reports by the AAMC on the composition of the physician workforce, with special attention to race and gender. All were published in Washington, DC, by the AAMC's Division of Diversity Policy and Programs under the title Diversity in the Physician Workforce: Facts & Figures, followed by the year, and are available online. I have used the reports covering the years 2000–2022. Some of the tables also include data starting in the 1970s that show changes over time.

2. AACM, *Diversity in the Physician Workforce* 2010, table 16a, 92. See also Gary King and Robert Bendel, "A Statistical Model for Estimating the Number of African American Physicians in the United Sates," *JNMA* 87 (April 1995): 264–72.

3. AACM, *Diversity in the Physician Workforce 2006*, tables 37 and 45, pp. 106, 116.

4. Montgomery, interview.

5. King and Bendel, "A Statistical Model Estimating the Number of African American Physicians in the United States," and AACM, *Diversity in Medical Education* 2000, figure 9, 23.

6. See Byrd and Clayton, *An American Health Dilemma*, 555–56; AACM, *Diversity in Medical Education* 2012, tables 2, 6, 8, pp. 58, 68, 72–74.

7. See Harriet A. Washington et al., "Segregation, Civil Rights, and Health Disparities: The Legacy of African American Physicians and Organized Medicine, 1910–1968," *JNMA* 101 (January 2009): 513–27.

8. Howell Raines, "Black Doctors Assert Race Is a Factor at Alabama Hospitals," *The New York Times*, April 22, 1979.

9. W. M. Byrd et al., "African American Physicians' Views on Health Reform: Results of a Survey," *JNMA*, 86 (March 1994): 191–99. See also *JNMA* 79 (October 1979): 1027–29, and Byrd and Clayton, *An American Health Dilemma*, 320–21, 414–15.

10. Damon Tweedy, *Black Man in a White Coat: A Doctor's Reflections on Race and Medicine* (New York: Picador ebook, 2015), 5, 12–13.

11. Kendal L. Foster, interview; and Underwood III, interview.

12. Janice Morton-Hunte, interview by Jack D. Ellis, Mobile, Alabama, October 22, 1998.

13. See James F. Adams and Ronald E. Jones, *Alabama Medicaid. Alabama Fiscal Year 1976*, plates 2, 4, 3, 7, 12, pp. 3, 6, 9. See also Rene P. McEldowney, "The Alabama Medicaid Reform Plan," in *Medicaid Reform and the American States: Studies in the Politics of Managed Care*, ed. Mark Ross Daniels (Westport, CT: Auburn House, 1998), 13–26.

14. James E. Cameron, "The Tallapoosa County Medical Society," *JMASA* 52 (July 1982): 22, online at Harvard Countway Library, State Medical Society Journals, Alabama.

15. *The Anniston Star*, May 2, 1979.

16. *The Montgomery Advertiser*, May 19, 1977; and Ira L. Myers, "Ecology of Health," *JMASA* 41 (July 1971): 53–54, 58, 65.

17. See Jessica Greene, Jan Blustein, and Beth W. Weitzman, "Race, Segregation, and Physicians' Participation in Medicaid," *The Milbank Quarterly: A Multidisciplinary Journal of Population Health and Health Policy* 84 (June 2006): 239–72. See also Frank Sloan, Janet B. Mitchell, and Jerry Cromwell, "Physician Participation in State Medicaid Programs," *The Journal of Human Resources* 13 (1978): 211–45; Janet B. Mitchell and Jerry Cromwell, "Large Medicaid Practices and Medicaid Mills," *JAMA* 244 (November 1980): 2433–37; Janet B. Mitchell, "Physician Participation in Medicaid Revisited," *Medical Care* 29 (July 1991): 645–53; and Janet D. Perloff, Phillip Kletke, and James M. Fossett, "Which Physicians Limit Their Medicaid Participation and Why," *HRS: Health Services Research* 30 (April 1995): 7–26.

18. House of Representatives, *Hearing before the Subcommittee on Health and the Environment*, September 8, 1990 (Washington, DC: US Government Printing Office, 1980), 29–36.

19. *The Anniston Star*, February 15, 1979; and January 9 and 28 May 1990.

20. *The Anniston Star*, February 15, 1979.

21. *The Montgomery Advertiser*, May 16, 1977.

22. L. C. Elam, "Meharry Looks Ahead," *JNMA* 61 (January 1969): 40–43. See also W. M. Byrd et al., "African American Physicians' Views on Health Reform: Results of a Survey," *JNMA* 86 (March 1994): 191–99.

23. See the *Birmingham Post-Herald*, March 15, 1977; and *The Montgomery Advertiser*, September 18, 1977.

24. *The Montgomery Advertiser*, July 17, 1975, and February 19, 1976.

25. Ronald E. Henderson, *The Tenant Farmer's Son: It's Not Where You End Up in Life, It's How Far You've Come* (Birmingham, AL: Twin Valley Press, 2015), 6, 102–08, 182–87.

26. For the full list of earners, including dentists, see *The Montgomery Advertiser*, February 11, 1977.

27. Rosemary Stevens and Robert Stevens, "Medicaid: Anatomy of a Dilemma," *Law and Contemporary Problems* 36 (Spring 1970): 348–425.

28. Joe McFadden in *The Montgomery Advertiser*, October 23, 1988.

29. See *The Montgomery Advertiser*, September 29,1987, and September 11, July 19, and October 23, 1988. See also *The Anniston Star*, July 14, 1988.

30. *The Anniston Star*, August 15 and October 4 1978, and April 1, 1983.

31. *The Montgomery Advertiser*, September 1, 1978.

32. See *The Anniston Star*, April 24, 1981, and March 10, 1982; and the *Montgomery Advertiser*, March 17, 1982.

33. For examples of press reports on these cases, see *Jet* magazine, February 9, 1967; the *Mobile Register*, January 9, 1976, and April 15, 1981; and *The Montgomery Advertiser*, April 7, 1989. See also Sidney Wolfe et al., *Questionable Doctors Disciplined*

by State and Federal Governments: Alabama, Georgia (Washington, DC: Public Citizen Health Research Group, 2000), AL-13–AL-14.

34. My thanks to Ron Hunter of the Alabama Board of Medical Examiners for providing this information.

35. Wolfe et al., *Questionable Doctors*, Al-1–Al-48.

36. See Henry N. Pontell et al., "A Demographic Portrait of Physicians Sanctioned by the Federal Government for Fraud and Abuse Against Medicare and Medicaid," *Medical Care 23* (August 1985): 1028–31.

37. Kaiser Family Foundation, State Health Facts, Poverty Rates by Race/Ethnicities, Alabama (2010), online.

38. David J. Becker and Michael A. Morrisey, "An Economic Evaluation of Medicaid Expansion in Alabama under the Affordable Care Act," Department of Health Care Organization and Policy, School of Public Health, University of Alabama at Birmingham (November 5, 2012), online.

39. See the FollowTheMoney (website), Medical Association of the State of Alabama (1996–2023), which lists amounts received from MASA by both Republican and Democratic candidates.

40. AACM 2021, "State Physician Workforce Data Report" (January 2022), 28–40.

41. Liliana M. Garces and David Mickey-Pabello, "Racial Diversity in the Medical Profession: The Impact of Affirmative Action Bans on Underrepresented Student of Color Matriculation in Medical Schools," *The Journal of Higher Education* 86 (March-April 2015): 264–94.

42. Miriam Komaromy, "The Role of Black and Hispanic Physicians in Providing Health Care for Underserved Populations," *The New England Journal of Medicine* 334 (16 May 1996): 1305–10.

43. Damon Tweedy, "The Case for Black Doctors," *The New York Times*, May 15, 2015.

44. See "Segregation, Civil Rights, and Health Disparities: The Legacy of African American Physicians and Organized Medicine, 1910–1968," *JNMA* 101 (2009): 513–27.

Bibliography

ARCHIVAL SOURCES

Alabama Department of Archives and History. Alabama State Board of Medical Examiners.

Application for certificate of qualification to practice medicine, 1879–1912. GR-BME-1.

Applications to practice medicine roster, 1875–1932. GR-BME-2

Examination questions, 1907–1969. GR-BME-6.

State and County Examination Tabulations, 1906-–1977. GR-BME-13.

University of Alabama at Birmingham Archives.

Jefferson County Medical Society Archives Reprint Files, MC53.

Office of the Dean, Medical College of Alabama, 1945–1969. Record Group 17.1.

ORAL HISTORIES

The forty oral histories used in this book are taken from a group of fifty-five completed between 1997 and 2004 that are now located in the University of Alabama at Birmingham Archives as the Jack D. Ellis Collection of Oral History Interviews with African American Physicians. The collection contains original cassette tapes plus annotated transcriptions. All interviews were conducted by Jack D. Ellis.

Barefield-Pendleton, Tyree James (1917–2010). Birmingham, Alabama. July, 20 1999.

Brewer, Alexander Lee (1915–2006). Birmingham, Alabama. July 21, 1999.

Calhoun, Calvin Lee (1927–2005). Nashville, Tennessee. October 8, 1998.

Calhoun, Thomas J. (1924–2000). Tuskegee, Alabama. October 15, 1998.

Carroll, Lawrence E. (1926–2000). Mobile, Alabama. October 22, 1998.

Curry, Dodson M. (1922–2018). Birmingham, Alabama. July 21, 1999.

Donalson, Claudia M. (1913–2007). Fayetteville, Tennessee. July 31, 1997.

Dowe, Calvin R. (1925–2004). Tuskegee, Alabama. October 15, 1998.

Dunn, Felix H. (1919–2002). Gulfport, Mississippi. October 20, 1998.

Forrester, J. L. B. (1912–2000). Nashville, Tennessee. October 1, 1998.

Foster, Alma W. (1925–2017). Mobile, Alabama. October 23, 1998.

Foster, Kendal I. (b. 1954). Mobile, Alabama. October 21, 1998.

Franklin, Marguerite W. (1906–2005). Mobile, Alabama. October 21, 1998.

Hansen, Axel Carl (1919–2008). Nashville, Tennessee. September 17, 1998.

Hereford, Sonnie Wellington, III (1931–2016). Huntsville, Alabama. Multiple interviews between 1997 and 2005.

Hume, John Franklin (1915–2004). Tuskegee, Alabama. October 14, 1998.

Hunte, Eyston A. (b. 1944). Mobile, Alabama. October 21, 1998.

Johns, Calvin R., Jr. (b. 1930). Montgomery, Alabama. October 21, 1998.

Johnson, Charles W. (1922–1999). Nashville, Tennessee. October 8, 1998.

Johnson, Charlotte E. (b. 1933). Alton, Illinois. Telephone interviews. July 17, 18, 2000.

Kates, William A. (1920–2012). Huntsville, Alabama. February 28, 2001.

LeFlore, Walker B. (1928–2001). Mobile, Alabama. October 23, 1998.

McGruder, Charles E. (1925–2015). Nashville, Tennessee. October 1,1998.

Montgomery, James T. (1925–2012). Birmingham, Alabama. October 23, 1998.

Moore, Hiram B. (1914–2005). South Pittsburg, Tennessee. August 22 and September 26, 1997, and July 9, 1999.

Morton-Hunte, Janice (b. 1954). Mobile, Alabama. October 22, 1998.

Northcross, David C., Jr. (1917–2016). Telephone interview from Atlanta. January 4, 2000.

Northcross, Ophelia Burnett (b. 1926). Telephone interview from Detroit. January 5, 2000.

Perry, L. O. P. (1923–2009). Nashville, Tennessee. October 7, 1998.

Rodgers, Gordon A., Jr. (1915–2007). Anniston, Alabama. March 7, 2000.

Sherrer, John William (1930–2012). Anniston, Alabama. March 7, 2000.

Swope, Hattie (1906–?). Morgan County, Alabama. February 29, 2000.

Tarlton, Gadson Jack, Jr. (1920–2022). Nashville, Tennessee. October 7, 1998.

Underwood, Jefferson, Jr. (1923–2011). Montgomery, Alabama. October 26, 1998.

Underwood, Jefferson, III (b. 1955). Montgomery, Alabama. October 26, 1998.

Walker, Charlotte (1938–2009). Nashville, Tennessee. September 17, 1998.

Wallace, Alfreda Swan (1942–2002). Telephone interview from Tuskegee. Alabama. July 30, 1999.

Whatley, Geneva Drake (1923–2007). Huntsville, Alabama. July 26, 1999.

Wilson, Hagalyn Seay (1930–2006). Montgomery, Alabama. October 27, 1998.

Winston, John H., Jr. (1928–2019). Montgomery, Alabama. October 26, 1998.

BIOGRAPHICAL DICTIONARIES AND ONLINE SOURCES

Beckford, Geraldine Rhoades. *Biographical Dictionary of American Physicians of African Ancestry, 1800–1920.* Cherry Hill, NJ: Africana Homestead Legacy Publishers, 2011.

Hamilton, Green Polonius. *Beacon Lights of the Race.* Memphis, TN: E. H. Clark and Brother, 1911.

Richardson, Clement, ed. *The National Cyclopedia of the Colored Race.* Vol. I. Montgomery, AL: National Publishing Company, 1919.

Sammons, Vivian Ovelton. *Blacks in Science and Medicine*. New York: Hemisphere Publishing Corporation, 1990.

Wright, A. J. *Hidden Legacies: I. Early African-American Physicians in Alabama*. Early African American Physicians in Alabama (website).

US CENSUS RECORDS

Social Explorer (website).

CORRESPONDENCE AND INTERVIEWS

Boulware, Thomas M., interview with Virginia Fisher. Birmingham, Alabama. June 30, 1987. UAB Archives, MC53, 4.15.

Brewer, Hampton, interview with William Bryant. City of Birmingham, *The Consortium. Concise History of Blacks in Medicine, 1983–84*. UAB Archives, MC53, 51/2.

Dinkins, William, interview with Blackside, Inc. September 17, 1979. *Eyes on the Prize: America's Civil Rights Years (1954–1965). Washington University Libraries, Film and Media Archive, Henry Hampton Collection*. Available at Washington University in St. Louis (website).

Harlan, Louis R., Raymond W. Smock, and Geraldine McTighe, eds. *The Booker T. Washington Papers*. Urbana: University of Illinois Press, 1972–1989.

Harriman, Joy HP. *Health Care in Mobile: An Oral History of the 1940s*. CreateSpace Independent Publishing Platform, 2011.

Heller, John R., interview with Wyndham D. Miles. Washington, D.C. October 26, 1964. National Institutes of Health (website).

Zukoski, Charles F. Jr., interview with Cliff Kuhn. September 13, 1984. University of Alabama Libraries Digital Archives. The University of Alabama Libraries (website).

GOVERNMENT PUBLICATIONS

US Department of Health and Human Services, Office of Inspector General. "Individuals Excluded from Participating in the Alabama Title XIX (Medicaid) Program." January 8, 2018. Alabama state government (website).

United States Commission on Civil Rights. *Title VI One Year After: A Survey of Desegregation of Health and Welfare Services in the South*, February 1966. The University of Maryland, Baltimore (website).

United States Court of Appeals, Fifth Circuit. *Maynard V Foster and LeBaron A. Foster v Mobile County Hospital Board et al.*, June 24, 1968, (CA5 Ala) 398 F2d 227, 37 ALR3d 637 *American Law Reports, Annotated Third Series*. Bancroft-Whitney Company, (1971): 637–44.

MEDICAL JOURNALS AND PUBLICATIONS

Association of American Medical Colleges (AAMC). *Diversity in the Physician Workforce: Facts & Figures*. Washington, DC, 2006, 2008, 2010, 2014, and 2016.

Association of American Medical Colleges (website).

Journal of the Medical Association of the State of Alabama. Montgomery: [the Association], 1931–1983. Harvard Library (website).

Journal of the National Medical Association 1909–2007. National Library of Medicine (website).

Medical Association of the State of Alabama, *Transactions.* Montgomery [the Association]: 1890–1973. Issues for 1866 to 1922 are available at HathiTrust (website).

NEWSPAPERS

Excluding microfilm collections consulted at the Birmingham and Huntsville public libraries, the following titles were cited from two online sources: Newspapers.com (website) and NewspaperArchive.com (asterisks denote Black newspapers).

The Anniston Star

The Birmingham News

Birmingham Post

Birmingham Post-Herald

**Birmingham World*

**The Chicago Defender*

The Cincinnati Enquirer

Detroit Free Press

The Huntsville Times

[Mobile] Press-Register

Montgomery Advertiser

**The Nashville Globe*

**The New York Age*

The New York Times

**The Pittsburgh Courier*

The Southern Courier, a Montgomery-based newspaper edited by a group of mostly white Harvard undergraduates who had come south during the 1960s to cover civil rights news ignored by the local press. May be found at *The Southern Courier* (website).

MEDICAL AND CIVIL RIGHTS MEMOIRS

Brummit, Houston. *Talladega Days. Race, Rural Life, and Memories of a Forgotten Legend and KKK Survivor.* Bloomington, IN.: iUniverse, 2011.

Cashin, Sheryll. *The Agitator's Daughter: A Memoir of Four Generations of One Extraordinary African-American Family.* New York: Perseus Books Group, 2008.

Chestnut, J. L., Jr., and Julia Cass. *Black in Selma: the Uncommon Life of J. L. Chestnut, Jr.* New York: Farrar, Straus and Giroux, 1990.

Conner, Douglas L., and John F. Marszalek. *A Black Physician's Story: Bringing Hope in Mississippi.* Jackson: University Press of Mississippi, 1985.

Eaton, Hubert A., Sr. *Everyman Should Try.* Wilmington, NC: Bonaparte Press, 1984.

Foster, Henry W., Jr., and Alice Greenwood. *Make a Difference.* New York: Scriber, 1997.

Garrow, David J., ed. *The Montgomery Bus Boycott and the Women Who Started It: The Memoir of Jo Ann Gibson Robinson*. Knoxville: University of Tennessee Press, 1987.

Gray, Fred. *Bus Ride to Justice: The Life and Works of Fred Gray*. Montgomery, AL: The Black Belt Press, 1995.

———. *The Tuskegee Syphilis Study: The Real Story and Beyond*. Montgomery, AL: NewSouth Books, 1998.

Hereford, Sonnie Wellington, III, and Jack D. Ellis. *Beside the Troubled Waters: A Black Doctor Remembers Life, Medicine, and Civil Rights in an Alabama Town*. Tuscaloosa: University of Alabama Press, 2011.

Jackson, Richie Jean Sherrod. *The House by the Side of the Road: The Selma Civil Rights Movement*. Tuscaloosa: University of Alabama Press, 2011.

Lee, Helen Shores, and Barbara S. Shores, *The Gentle Giant of Dynamite Hill: The Untold Story of Arthur Shores and His Family's Fight for Civil Rights*. Grand Rapids, MI: Zondervan, 2012.

Lewis, John, and Michael D'Orso. *Walking with the Wind: A Memoir of the Movement*. New York: Simon & Schuster, 1998.

Lofton, J. Mack, Jr. *Healing Hands: An Alabama Medical Mosaic*. Tuscaloosa and London: University of Alabama Press, 1995.

Logan, Onnie Lee, and Katherine Clark. *Motherwit: An Alabama Midwife's Story*. New York: E. P. Dutton, 1989.

Manis, Andrew Michael. *A Fire You Can't Put Out: The Civil Rights Life of Birmingham's Reverend Fred Shuttlesworth*. Tuscaloosa: University of Alabama Press, 1999.

Mason, Gilbert R., and James Patterson Smith. *Beaches, Blood, and Ballots: A Black Doctor's Civil Rights Struggle*. Jackson: University Press of Mississippi, 2000.

Noble, Phil. *Beyond the Burning Bus: The Civil Rights Revolution in a Southern Town*. Montgomery, AL: NewSouth Books, 2011.

Norris, James E. C. *Fight On, My Soul: A Colored Doctor's Battle Against Disease, Discrimination, and Ignorance in Rural Jim Crow Virginia*. Pella, IA: The Write Place, 2009.

Power (Chappell), Edith, and John F. Hume. *A Black Oasis: Tuskegee Institute's Fight Against Infantile Paralysis*. March of Dimes Birth Defects Foundation, 1987.

Quigless, Dr. Milton D., Sr. *Looking Back—The Way Things Were: The Autobiography of Dr. Milton D. Quigless Sr.* Nashville, TN.: C2 Printing & Design, 1994.

Ridlon, Florence. *A Black Physician's Struggle for Civil Rights: Edward C. Mazique, M.D.* Albuquerque: University of New Mexico Press, 2005.

Rosengarten, Theodore. *All God's Dangers: The Life of Nate Shaw*. New York: Vintage Books, 1974.

Seay, Solomon S., Sr. *I Was There by the Grace of God: An Autobiography Written in Fulfillment of a Request by Dr. Martin Luther King, Jr.* Montgomery, AL: The S. S. Seay Sr. Educational Foundation, 1990.

Smith, Margaret Charles, and Linda Janet Holmes. *Listen to Me Good: The Life Story of an Alabama Midwife*. Columbus: Ohio State University Press, 1996.

Tarry, Ellen. *The Third Door: the Autobiography of an American Negro Woman*. New

York: David McKay Company, 1955.

Tweedy, Damon. *Black Man in a White Coat: A Doctor's Reflections on Race and Medicine*. New York: Picador ebook, 2015.

Webb, Sheyann, and Rachel West Nelson. *Selma, Lord, Selma: Girlhood Memories of the Civil Rights Days*. Tuscaloosa: University of Alabama Press, 1980.

Wells, Clay Norris. *Please God, Don't Call Me to Preach*. New York: iUniverse, Inc., 2004.

Wilkerson, E. L. *Struggling to Climb: A Biography*. Cleveland, Ohio: Carpenter Printing Co., 1958.

Witt, Edwin T. *Witt's End*. Victorville, CA.: E&C Publishers, 1996.

Young, Andrew. *An Easy Burden: The Civil Rights Movement and the Transformation of America*. New York: HarperCollins, 1996.

CONTEMPORARY MEDICAL WRITINGS

American Medical Association. "Medical Licensure Statistics for 1946." *JAMA* 134 (May 1946): 255–69.

Bent, Michael J., and Ellen F. Greene. *Rural Negro Health: A Report on a Five-Year Experiment in Health Education in Tennessee*. Nashville, TN: Julius Rosenwald Fund, 1937.

Boulware, T. M., Elizabeth LaForge, and R. C. Stewart. "A Negro Demonstration Center for Maternal and Newborn Care in Alabama." *Southern Medical Journal* 36 (1943): 748–91.

Bousfield, M. O. "Internships, Residencies and Postgraduate Training." *JNMA* 32 (January 1940): 24–30.

Brown, Roscoe C. "The National Negro Health Week Movement." *The Journal of Negro Education* 6 (July 1937): 553–64.

Callis, H. A. "The Need and Training of Negro Physicians." *Journal of Negro Education* 4 (January 1935): 32–41.

Chenault, John W. "The Crippled Child." *JNMA* 28 (August 1936): 124–26.

Cornely, Paul B. "Distribution of Negro Physicians in the United States in 1942." *JAMA* 124 (March 1944): 826–30.

Crowley, Anne E., and Hayden C. Nicholson. "The Education of Negroes for Medicine." *JNMA* 61 (September 1969): 375–81.

Dibble, Eugene H., Louis A. Rabb, and Ruth B. Ballard. "John A. Andrew Memorial Hospital." *JNMA* 51 (March 1961): 103–18.

Dummett, Clifton O. and Eugene H. Dibble [Jr.]. "Historical Notes on the Tuskegee Veterans Hospital." *JNMA* 54 (March 1962): 133–38.

Frazier, Edward Franklin. "The Pathology of Race Prejudice." *The Forum* 77 (June 1927): 856–62.

Frazier, William H. "Negro School Children in Tuskegee: Their Health and Their Environment." *Opportunity: A Journal of Negro Life* 13 (December 1935): 360–63.

———. "The Rural Negro Physician." *Opportunity: A Journal of Negro Life* 15 (March 1937): 79–81.

Harris, Seale. "The Future of the Negro from the Standpoint of the Southern Physician." *The Alabama Medical Journal* 14 (January 1902): 57–68.

Haynes, M. Alfred. "The Distribution of Black Physicians in the United States, 1967." *JNMA* 61 (November 1969): 470–73.

Kenney, Howard W., and Julian W. Giles. "Tuskegee Veterans Administration Hospital—Present and Future." *JNMA* 54 (March 1962): 139–45.

Kenney, John A. *The Negro in Medicine.* Marietta, GA: Harper House Publishers, 2008.

———. "A Brief History of the Origin of the John A. Andrew Clinics by the Founder." *JNMA* 26 (May 1934): 65–68.

———. "Despise Not the Day of Small Beginnings." *JNMA* 38 (July 1946): 127–32.

———. "The First Graduating Class of the Tuskegee School of Midwifery," *JNMA* 34 (May 1942): 107–9.

———. "The Late Booker T. Washington: Friend of the Negro Physician." *JNMA* (November 1946): 225–26.

———. "Second Annual Oration on Surgery: The Negro's Contribution to Surgery." *JNMA 33* (September 1941): 203–14.

———. "Our Hospital: A Factor in the Prevention and Treatment of Disease." *JNMA* 5 (April-June 1913): 77–81.

Maddux, Walter H. "The Slossfield Health Center: An Example of Local Medical Service for Mothers and Children under Public Health Auspices." *American Journal of Public Health* 31 (May 1941): 481–86.

"Malaria in Alabama: Prevalence and Geographic Distribution—1915 and 1916." *Public Health Reports (1896–1970)* 32 (21 December 1917): 2165–68.

Odom, Earl T. "Medical Resident Training Program, Veterans Administration Hospital, Tuskegee, Alabama." *JNMA* 54 (March 1962): 146–48.

Taylor, C. F., ed. "The Colored Physicians Speak in their Defense." *The Medical World: A Practical Medical Monthly* 32 (March 1914): 111–13.

Walcott, B. B. "Alabama Heals Her Crippled Children." *The Crisis* (February 1940): 47, 62.

Walker, Alfred A. et al. *A Report of the Jefferson County Board of Health Covering the Years 1943 and 1944* (August 1945). UAB Archives, MC53, 5.35.

Washington, Booker T. "The Negro Doctor in the South." In *Booker T. Washington Rediscovered*, edited by Michael Scott Bieze and Marybeth Gasman, 104–6. Baltimore, MD: The Johns Hopkins Press, 2012.

West, A. E. "Surgery in the Rural Districts: Some Helpful Hints." *JNMA* 10 (January–March 1918): 25–31.

Wilkerson, Robert S. "The Residency Training Program in General Surgery, Tuskegee Veterans Administration Hospital." *JNMA* 54 (March 1962): 149–51.

Yancey, Asa, "The Surgical Residency Programs at the Tuskegee VA Hospital and the Hughes Spalding Pavilion, Atlanta: With Twelve Case Reports." *JNMA* 54 (March 1962): 166–73.

JOURNAL ARTICLES AND BOOK CHAPTERS

Beardsley, Edward H. "Goodbye to Jim Crow: The Desegregation of Southern Hospitals, 1945–70." *Bulletin of the History of Medicine* 60 (1986): 367–86.

———. "Making Separate, Equal: Black Physicians and the Problems of Medical Segregation in the Pre-World War II South." *Bulletin of the History of Medicine* 57 (Fall 1983): 382–96.

Byrd, W. Michael, and Linda A. Clayton. "Race, Medicine, and Health Care in the United States: A Historical Survey." *JNMA* 93 (March 2001): 11S–27S.

Byrd, W. Michael et al. "African American Physicians' Views on Health Reform: Results of a Survey." *JNMA* 86 (March 1994): 191–99.

———. "Inquisition, Peer Review, and Black Physician Survival." *JNMA* 79 (October 1987): 1027–29.

Charatz-Litt, Cynthia. "A Chronicle of Racism: the Effects of the White Medical Community on Black Health." *JNMA* 84 (August 1992): 717–25.

Coelhol, Philip R. P., and Robert A. McGuire. "Racial Differences in Disease Susceptibilities: Intestinal Worm Infections in the Early Twentieth-Century American South." *Social History of Medicine* 19 (December 2006): 461–82.

"Current Practice Characteristics and Distribution Patterns of Alabama Physicians." *Journal of the Medical Association of the State of Alabama* 52 (May 1983): 22–27.

Dorr, Gary Michael. "Defective or Disabled?: Race, Medicine, and Eugenics in Progressive Era Virginia and Alabama." *Journal of the Gilded Age and Progressive Era* 5 (October 2006): 359–92.

Dummett, Clifton Orrin. "Dentistry's Beginnings among Blacks in the United States." *JNMA* 66 (July 1974): 321–27.

———. "Dentistry, Too, in Patient Care at Tuskegee." *JNMA* 54 (March 1962): 162–65.

———. "Homage to the NMA: The NDA Story (1895–1975)—Part 1." *JNMA* 89 (July 1997): 486–92.

———. "Homage to the NMA: The NDA Story (1895–1975)—Part 2." *JNMA* 89 (August 1997): 555–63.

Epps, Howard R. "The Howard University Medical Department in the Flexner Era: 1910–1929." *JNMA* 81 (August 1989): 885–911.

Flynt, Wayne. "Alabama's Shame: The Historical Origins of the 1901 Constitution." *Alabama Law Review* 53 (2001): 67–76.

Garces, Liliana M., and David Mickey-Pabello. "Racial Diversity in the Medical Profession: The Impact of Affirmative Action Bans on Underrepresented Student of Color Matriculation in Medical Schools." *The Journal of Higher Education* 86 (March–April 2015): 264–94.

Goldenberg, Robert L. "Maternal and Child Health in Alabama." *Journal of the Medical Association of the State of Alabama* 48 (March 1979): 13–16, 28–29, 44.

Greene, Jessica, Jan Blustein, and Beth C. Weitzman. "Race, Segregation, and Physicians' Participation in Medicaid." *The Milbank Quarterly: A Multidisciplinary Journal of Population Health and Health Policy* 84 (June 2006): 239–72.

Hall, Jacquelyn Dowd. "The Long Civil Rights Movement and the Political Uses of the Past." *The Journal of American History* 91 (March 2005): 1233–63.

Hasson, Gail S. "Health and Welfare of Freedmen in Reconstruction Alabama." *Alabama Review* 35 (April 1982): 94–110.

Houde, John B., Beverly W. Boyd, and Robert L. Goldenberg. "Out of Hospital Deliveries in Alabama 1940–1980." *Journal of the Medical Association of the State of Alabama* 52 (August 1982): 20–25.

King, Gary, and Robert Bendel. "A Statistical Model Estimating the Number of African American Physicians in the United States." *JNMA* 87 (April 1995): 264–72.

Klapper, Margaret S. "The Alabama Experience in Minority Recruitment." *JNMA* 65 (July 1973): 322–26.

Komaromy, Miriam. "The Role of Black and Hispanic Physicians in Providing Health Care for Underserved Populations." *The New England Journal of Medicine* 334 (May 1996): 1305–1310.

McEldowney, René P. "The Alabama Medicaid Reform Plan." In *Medicaid Reform and the American States: Studies in the Politics of Managed Care,* edited by Mark Ross Daniels, 13–26. Westport, CT: Auburn House, 1998.

Mitchell, Janet B., and Jerry Cromwell. "Large Medicaid Practices and Medicaid Mills." *JAMA* 244 (November 1980): 2433–37.

Mitchell, Janet B. "Physician Participation in Medicaid Revisited." *Medical Care* 29 (July 1991): 645–53.

Nelson, Jennifer. "Healthcare Reconsidered: Forging Community Wellness among African Americans in the South." *Bulletin of the History of Medicine* 81 (Fall 2007): 594–624.

Perloff, Janet D., Phillip Kletke, and James M. Fossett. "Which Physicians Limit Their Medicaid Participation and Why." *HRS: Health services Research* 30 (April 1995): 7–26.

Rao, Vijaya, and Glenn Flores. "Why Aren't There More African-American Physicians? A Qualitative Study and Exploratory Inquiry of African American Students' Perspectives on Careers in Medicine." *JNMA* 99 (September 2007): 986–93.

Reede, Joan Y. "A Recurring Theme: The Need for Minority Physicians." *Health Affairs* 22 (2003): 91–93.

Reynolds, P. Preston. "Hospitals and Civil Rights, 1945–1963: The Case of *Simkins v Moses H. Cone Memorial Hospital.*" *Annals of Internal Medicine* 126 (June 1997): 898–906.

Rice, Mitchell F., and Woodrow Jones Jr. "Black Health Inequities and the American Health Care System." *Health Policy and Education* 3 (1982): 195–214.

———. "The Hill-Burton Act and Black Hospitals." In *Public Policy and the Black Hospital: From Slavery to Segregation to Integration.* Westport, CT.: Greenwood Press, 1994: 73–100.

Rogers, Naomi. "Race and the Politics of Polio: Warm Springs, Tuskegee, and the March of Dimes." *American Journal of Public Health* 97 (May 2007): 784–96.

Savitt, Todd L. "The Invisible Malady: Sickle Cell Anemia in America: 1910–1970." *Journal of the National Medical Association* 73 (August 1981): 739–746.

———. "The Education of Physicians at Shaw University, 1882–1918: Problems of

Quality and Quantity." In *Black Americans in North Carolina and the South*, edited by Jeffrey Crow and Flora J. Hatley, 160–188. Chapel Hill: University of North Carolina Press, 1984.

———. "Lincoln University Medical Department: A Forgotten Black Medical School." *Journal of the History of Medicine and Allied Sciences* 40 (1985): 42–65.

———. "Entering a White Profession: Black Physicians in the New South, 1880–1920." *Bulletin of the History of Medicine* 61 (1987): 507–540

———. "Four African-American Proprietary Medical Colleges: 1888–1923." *Journal of the History of Medicine* 55 (July 2000): 203–53.

———. "Abraham Flexner and the Black Medical Schools." In *Flexner and the 1990s: Medical Education in the 20th Century*, edited by Barbara M. Barzansky and Norman Gevitz, 65–81. Westport, CT: Greenwood Press, 1992.

Schwarz, George E., and Montague S. Lawrence. "Selected Characteristics of the National Medical Association: Preliminary Findings." *JNMA* 62 (January 1970): 1–8.

Sloan, Frank, Janet B. Mitchell, and Jerry Cromwell. "Physician Participation in State Medicaid Programs." *The Journal of Human Resources* 13 (1978): 211–45.

Smith, Susan L. "Neither Victim Nor Villain: Eunice Rivers, the Tuskegee Syphilis Experiment, and Public Health Work." *Journal of Women's History* 8 (Spring 1996): 95–113.

Stevens, Robert B. "Medicaid: Anatomy of a Dilemma." (1970). *Faculty Scholarship Series*. Paper 4188. Yale Law School (website).

Verney, Kevin. "'To Hope Till Hope Creates': The NAACP in Alabama, 1913–1945." In *Long Is the Way and Hard: One Hundred Years of the National Association for the Advancement of Colored People (NAACP)*, edited by Kevern Verney and Lee Sartain, 105–20. Fayetteville: University of Arkansas Press, 2000.

Wall, Barbra Mann. "Catholic Sister Nurses in Selma, Alabama, 1940–1972." *Advances in Nursing Science* 32 (January–March 2009): 91–102.

Washington, Harriet A. et al. "Segregation, Civil Rights, and Health Disparities: The Legacy of African American Physicians and Organized Medicine, 1910–1968." *JNMA* 101 (January 2009): 513–27.

White, Robert M. "Misrepresentations of the Tuskegee Study of Untreated Syphilis." *JNMA* 97 (December 2005): 1729–31.

———. "Unraveling the Tuskegee Study of Untreated Syphilis." *Archives of Internal Medicine* 13 (March 2000): 585–98.

Willard, William R., Elizabeth R. Ruben, and Harry J. Knopke. "Current Practice Characteristics and Distribution Patterns of Alabama Physicians." *Journal of the Medical Association of the State of Alabama* 52 (May 1983): 22–27.

BOOKS AND MONOGRAPHS

Alexander, Shawn Leigh. *An Army of Lions: The Civil Rights Struggle before the NAACP*. Philadelphia: University of Pennsylvania Press, 2012.

Anderson, James D. *The Education of Blacks in the South*. Chapel Hill and London: University of North Carolina Press, 1988.

Barbeau, Arthur E., and Florette Henri. *The Unknown Soldiers: Black American Troops in World War I.* Philadelphia: Temple University Press, 1974.

Beardsley, Edward H. *A History of Neglect: Health Care for Blacks and Mill Workers in the Twentieth-Century South.* Knoxville: University of Tennessee Press, 1987.

Blackmon, Douglas A. *Slavery by Another Name: the Re-Enslavement of Black Americans from the Civil War to World War II.* New York: Anchor Books, 2009.

Bond, Horace Mann. *Negro Education in Alabama: A Study in Cotton and Steel.* In *Studies in American Negro Life,* edited by August Meier. New York: Atheneum, 1969.

Bornat, Joanna, Robert Perks, Paul Thompson, and Jan Walmsley, eds. *Oral History, Health and Welfare.* London and New York: Routledge, 2000.

Byrd, W. Michael, and Linda A Clayton. *An American Health Dilemma: Race, Medicine, and Health Care in the United States, 1900–2000.* New York and London: Routledge, 2002.

Carter, Dan T. *The Politics of Rage: George Wallace, the Origins of the New Conservatism, and the Transformation of American Politics.* New York: Simon & Schuster, 1995.

———. *Scottsboro: A Tragedy of the American South.* Baton Rouge: Louisiana State University Press, 1970.

Collins, Donald E. *When the Church Bell Rang Racist: The Methodist Church and the Civil Rights Movement in Alabama.* Macon, GA: Mercer University Press, 1998.

Connerly, Charles E. *"The Most Segregated City in America": City Planning and Civil Rights in Birmingham.* Charlottesville and London: University of Virginia Press, 2005.

Davis-Horton, Paulette. *Avenue . . . The Place, the People, the Memories.* Mobile, AL: Horton, 1991.

deShazo, Richard D., ed. *The Racial Divide in American Medicine.* Jackson, MS: University Press of Mississippi, 2018.

Dittmer, John. *Local People: The Struggle for Civil Rights in Mississippi.* Urbana: University of Illinois Press, 1995.

———. *The Good Doctors: The Medical Committee for Human Rights and the Struggle for Social Justice in Heath Care.* New York: Bloomsbury Press, 2009.

Downs, Jim. *Sick from Freedom: African-American Illness and Suffering during the Civil War and Reconstruction.* Oxford and New York: Oxford University Press, 2012.

Dubois, W. E. B. *The Health and Physique of the Negro American.* Atlanta, GA: Atlanta University Press, 1906.

Dummett, Clifton Orrin. *The Growth and Development of the Negro in Dentistry in the United States.* Chicago, IL: Stanek Press, 1952.

———. "Dentistry's Beginnings among Blacks in the United States." *JNMA* 66 (July 1974): 321–27.

———."Homage to the NMA: The NDA Story (1895–1975)—Part 1." *JNMA* 89 (July 1997): 486–92.

———. "Homage to the NMA: The NDA Story (1895–1975)—Part 2." *JNMA* 89 (August 1997): 555–63.

Egerton, John. *Speak Now Against the Day: The Generation before the Civil Rights Movement in the South.* New York: Alfred A. Knopf, 1994.

Eskew, Glenn T. *But for Birmingham: The Local and National Movements in the Civil Rights Struggle.* Chapel Hill: University of North Carolina Press, 1997.

Fabre, Geneviève Fabre, and Robert O'Meally, eds. *History and Memory in African-American Culture.* New York and Oxford: Oxford University Press, 1999.

Fallin, Wilson, Jr. *The African American Church in Birmingham, Alabama, 1815–1963: A Shelter in the Storm.* New York and London: Garland Publishing, 1997.

Fassin, Didier. *l'Espace politique de la santé: Essai de généalogie.* Paris: Presses Universitaires de France, 1996.

Feldman, Lynne B. *A Sense of Place: Birmingham's Black Middle-Class Community, 1890–1930.* Tuscaloosa and London: University of Alabama Press, 1999.

Flint, Wayne. *Poor but Proud: Alabama's Poor Whites.* Tuscaloosa and London: University of Alabama Press, 1989.

Fraser, Gertrude Jacinta. *African American Midwifery in the South: Dialogues of Birth, Race, and Memory.* Cambridge, MA: Harvard University Press, 1998.

Gaillard, Frye. *Cradle of Freedom: Alabama and the Movement That Changed America.* Tuscaloosa: University of Alabama Press, 2004.

Gamble, Vanessa Northington. *Making A Place for Ourselves: The Black Hospital Movement 1920–1945.* New York and Oxford: Oxford University Press, 1995.

Goldsmith, Jewell S., and Helen D. Fulton. *Medicine Bags and Bumpy Roads: A Heritage of Healing in Madison County, Town and County.* Huntsville, AL.: Valley Publishing, 1985.

Hine, Darlene Clark. *Black Women in White: Racial Conflict and Cooperation in the Nursing Profession 1890–1950.* Bloomington and Indianapolis: Indiana University Press, 1989.

Hoffman, Beatrix. *Health Care for Some: Rights and Rationing in the United States since 1930.* Chicago: University of Chicago Press, 2012.

Holley, Howard L. *A History of Medicine in Alabama.* Birmingham: University of Alabama School of Medicine, 1982.

Horsman, Reginald. *Josiah Nott of Mobile: Southerner, Physician, and Racial Theorist.* Baton Rouge: Louisiana State University Press, 1978.

Huntley, Horace, and John W. McKerley, eds. *Foot Soldiers for Democracy: The Men, Women, and Children of the Birmingham Civil Rights Movement.* Urbana and Chicago: University of Illinois Press, 2009.

Johnson, Charles Spurgeon. *Into the Main Stream: A Survey of the Best Practices in Race Relations in the South.* Chapel Hill: University of North Carolina Press, 1947.

Johnson, Charles W., Sr. *The Spirit of a Place Called Meharry: The Strength of Its Past to Shape Its Future.* Franklin, TN.: Hillsboro Press, 2000.

Johnson, Daniel M., and Rex R. Campbell. *Black Migration in America: A Social Demographic History.* Durham, NC: Duke University Press, 1981.

Johnson, Robert S. *Shadow of the Plantation.* Chicago: University of Chicago Press, 1934.

———. *Growing Up in the Black Belt: Negro Youth in the Rural South.* New York:

Schocken Books, 1941.

Jones, James H. *Bad Blood: The Tuskegee Syphilis Experiment.* New York: The Free Press, 1993.

Kaplan, Mary. *The Tuskegee Veterans Hospital and Its Black Physicians: The Early Years.* Jefferson, NC: McFarland & Company, 2016.

Kelley, Robin D. G. *Hammer and Hoe: Alabama Communists during the Great Depression.* Chapel Hill and London: University of North Carolina Press, 2015.

Koehlinger, Amy L. *The New Nuns: Racial Justice and Religious Reform in the 1960s.* Cambridge and London: Harvard University Press, 2007.

Kornweibel, Theodore. *"Investigate Everything": Federal Efforts to Compel Black Loyalty during World War I.* Bloomington: Indiana University Press, 2002.

LaMonte, Edward Shannon. *Politics & Welfare in Birmingham, 1900–1975.* Tuscaloosa and London: University of Alabama Press, 1995.

Levinson, Cynthia. *We've Got a Job: The 1963 Birmingham Children's March.* Atlanta, GA: Peachtree Publishers, 2012.

Long, Gretchen, *Doctoring Freedom: The Politics of African American Medical Care in Slavery and Emancipation.* Chapel Hill: University of North Carolina Press, 2012.

Love, Spencie. *One Blood: The Death and Resurrection of Charles R. Drew.* Chapel Hill: University of North Carolina Press, 1996.

Lovett, Bobby L. *The Civil Rights Movement in Tennessee: A Narrative History.* Knoxville: University of Tennessee Press, 2005.

McGregor, Deborah Kuhn. *Sexual Surgery and the Origins of Gynecology: J. Marion Sims, His Hospital, and His Patients.* New York and London: Garland Publishing, 1989.

McWilliams, Tennant S. *New Lights in the Valley: The Emergence of UAB.* Tuscaloosa: University of Alabama Press, 2007.

Mendelsohn, Jack. *The Martyrs: Sixteen Who Gave Their Lives for Racial Justice.* New York: Harper and Row, 1966.

Morrison, Melanie S. *Murder on Shades Mountain: The Legal Lynching of Willie Patterson and the Struggle for Justice in Jim Crow Birmingham.* Durham and London: Duke University Press, 2018.

Norrell, Robert J. *Reaping the Whirlwind: The Civil Rights Movement in Tuskegee.* New York: Alfred A. Knopf, 1985.

———. *Up from History: The Life of Booker T. Washington.* Cambridge, MA: Harvard University Press, 2009.

Nora, Pierre. *Les Lieux de Mémoires, I: La République.* Paris: Gallimard, 1984.

Organ, Claude H., Jr., and Margaret M. Kosiba, eds. *A Century of Black Surgeons: The USA Experience.* Vol. I. Norman, OK.: Transcript Press, 1987.

Patterson, James T. *Brown v. Board of Education: A Civil Rights Milestone and its Troubled Legacy.* Oxford and New York: Oxford University Press, 2001.

Pearson, Hugh. *Under the Knife: How a Wealthy Negro Surgeon Wielded Power in the Jim Crow South.* New York: The Free Press, 2000.

Pollitt, Phoebe Ann. *African American and Cherokee Nurses in Appalachia: A History, 1900–1965.* Jefferson, NC: McFarland & Company, 2016.

———.*African American Hospitals in North Carolina: 39 Institutional Histories*. Jefferson, NC: McFarland & Company, 2017.

Reverby, Susan M., ed. *Tuskegee's Truths: Rethinking the Tuskegee Syphilis Study*. Chapel Hill: University of North Carolina Press, 2000.

———.*Examining Tuskegee: The Infamous Syphilis Study and its Legacy*. Chapel Hill: University of North Carolina Press, 2009.

Richardson, Joe M., and Maxine D. Jones. *Education for Liberation: The American Missionary Association and African Americans, 1890 to the Civil Rights Movement*. Tuscaloosa: University of Alabama Press, 2009.

Robertson, Nancy Marie. *Christian Sisterhood, Race Relations, and the YWCA, 1906–46*. Urbana and Chicago: University of Illinois Press, 2007.

Rogers, William Warren, Robert David Ward, Leah Rawls Atkins, and Wayne Flynt. *Alabama: The History of a Deep South State*. Tuscaloosa: University of Alabama Press, 1994.

Savitt, Todd L. *Medicine and Slavery: The Diseases and Health Care of Blacks in Antebellum Virginia*. Urbana: University of Illinois Press, 1978.

Scribner, Christopher MacGregor. *Renewing Birmingham: Federal Funding and the Promise of Change, 1929–1979*. Athens and London: University of Georgia Press, 2002.

Sikora, Frank. *The Judge: The Life & Opinions of Alabama's Frank M. Johnson, Jr.* Montgomery, AL: Black Belt Press, 1992.

Smedley, Brian D., Adrienne Stith Butler, and Lonnie R. Bristow, eds. *In the Nation's Best Interest: Ensuring Diversity in the Health-Care Workforce*. Washington, DC: National Academies Press, 2004.

Smith, David Barton. *Health Care Divided: Race and Healing A Nation*. Ann Arbor: University of Michigan Press, 1999.

———. *The Power to Heal: Civil Rights, Medicare, and the Struggle to Transform America's Health Care System Nashville*. Nashville, TN: Vanderbilt University Press, 2016.

———. *The Forensic Case Files: Diagnosing and Treating the Pathologies of the American Health Care System*. Toh Tuck Link, Singapore: World Scientific Publishing CO., 2010.

Smith, Susan L. *Sick and Tired of Being Sick and Tired: Black Women's Health Activism in American, 1890–1950*. Philadelphia: University of Pennsylvania Press, 1995.

Stanton, Mary. *From Selma to Sorrow: The Life and Death of Viola Liuzzo*. Athens: University of Georgia Press, 1998.

Summerville, James. *Educating Black Doctors: A History of Meharry Medical College*. Tuscaloosa; University of Alabama Press, 1983.

Sweeney, W. Allison. *History of the American Negro in the Great World War*. New York: Negro Universities Press, 1919.

Thomas, Karen Kruse. *Deluxe Jim Crow: Civil Rights and American Health Policy, 1935–1954*. Athens and London: University of Georgia Press, 2011.

Thornton, J. Mills, III. *Dividing Lines: Municipal Politics and the Struggle for Civil Rights in Montgomery, Birmingham, and Selma*. Tuscaloosa and London:

University of Alabama Press, 2002.

Valk, Anne, and Leslie Brown. *Living with Jim Crow: African American Women and Memories of the Segregated South.* New York: Palgrave Macmillan, 2010.

Walker, Helen Edith. *The Negro in the Medical Profession.* Charlottesville: University of Virginia Press, 1949.

Ward, Thomas J., Jr. *Black Physicians in the Jim Crow South.* Fayetteville: University of Arkansas Press, 2003.

———. *Out in the Rural: A Mississippi Health Center & Its War on Poverty.* New York: Oxford University Press, 2017.

Watson, Wilbur H. *Against the Odds: Blacks in the Profession of Medicine in the United States.* New Brunswick and London: Transaction Publishers, 1999.

Winn, J. Emmett. *Documenting Racism: African Americans in US Department of Agriculture Documentaries, 1921–42.* New York: Continuum International Publishing Group, 2012.

Wolfe, Sidney, Phyllis McCarthy, Alana Bame, and Benita Marcus Adler. *Questionable Doctors Disciplined by State and Federal Governments: Alabama, Georgia.* Washington, DC: Public Citizen Health Research Group, 2000.

Index

Names in italics are those of African American physicians who passed their medical licensure examinations in Alabama and practiced in the state between 1877 and 1970. Page numbers referring to illustrations and maps also appear in italics.